Inside Chronic Pain

A VOLUME IN THE SERIES

The Culture and Politics of Health Care Work

edited by Suzanne Gordon and Sioban Nelson

A list of titles in the series is available at www.cornellpress.cornell.edu.

Inside
Chronic Pain

AN INTIMATE AND
CRITICAL ACCOUNT

LOUS HESHUSIUS

With a Clinical Commentary
by **Scott M. Fishman, MD**

Foreword by **David B. Morris**

ILR Press
an imprint of
Cornell University Press
Ithaca and London

First published 2009 by Cornell University Press

Printed in the United States of America

Library of Congress Cataloging-in-Publication Data

Heshusius, Lous.
   Inside chronic pain : an intimate and critical account / Lous Heshusius ; with a
clinical commentary by Scott M. Fishman ; foreword by David B. Morris.
       p. cm. — (The culture and politics of health care work)
   Includes bibliographical references and index.
   ISBN 978-0-8014-4796-9 (cloth : alk. paper)
   1. Chronic pain.   2. Chronic pain—Treatment.   I. Fishman, Scott, 1959–
II. Title.   III. Series: Culture and politics of health care work.
   RB127.H47   2009
   616'.0472—dc22   2009010907

Cornell University Press strives to use environmentally responsible suppliers
and materials to the fullest extent possible in the publishing of its books. Such
materials include vegetable-based, low-VOC inks and acid-free papers that are
recycled, totally chlorine-free, or partly composed of nonwood fibers. For further
information, visit our website at www.cornellpress.cornell.edu.

Cloth printing   10 9 8 7 6 5 4 3 2 1

A modern chronicler of hell might look to the lives of chronic pain patients for inspiration.

—MELANIE THERNSTROM, *Pain, the Disease*

The act of verbally expressing pain is a necessary prelude to the collective task of diminishing pain.

—ELAINE SCARRY, *The Body in Pain*

Though we want to be neutral in our feelings toward patients, we'll admit among ourselves that chronic-pain patients are a source of frustration and annoyance: presenting a malady we can neither explain nor alleviate, they shake our claims to competence and authority. We're all too happy to have [a pain specialist] take these patients off our hands.

—ATUL GAWANDE, *Complications: A Surgeon's Notes on an Imperfect Science*

Contents

Note from the Series Editors

In 2008 two books appeared with the title *How Doctors Think*. One was written by Jerome Groopman, a *New Yorker* writer and oncologist. Groopman's book appealed to a popular audience of patients and their families and became a bestseller. The other, by Kathryn Montgomery, a professor of medical humanities, was subtitled *Clinical Judgment and the Practice of Medicine* and addressed a more scholarly audience.

As soon as I heard about these new books, my first thought was, great, it's really important for patients to know how doctors think. My second was, what about doctors learning how patients think? As patients we have lots to say that would be beneficial not only to other patients but also to our doctors, nurses, and anyone else who cares for us when we are most vulnerable. Indeed, there is a vast literature of narratives that catalogue patient encounters—often more like collisions—with the medical system and those who practice within it. But how many doctors and other caregivers ever read these narratives? Reflecting on this, we tried to think of ways that these narratives by patients who have suffered in the system might have more value and reach a clinical audience as well as a popular one. In the end, we decided to present the patient's thought processes and experiences in a novel way that combines rather than counterposes the patient's and clinician's perspective by bringing them together in one book. This book—the story of a woman whose chronic pain has made her an expert patient—is the first in a new collection to be published under the rubric "How Patients Think" within our series The Culture and Politics of Health Care Work.

In this collection we will ask clinicians to listen, reflect, and learn from patients and describe how they—as doctors, nurses, or others—respond to the experiences of those they care for. In fact, we will bring together not just two but actually three points of view. Each book will be introduced with a foreword by a nonclinical observer of the medical system and those who work in it. This person is likely to be a medical sociologist, anthropologist, ethnographer, or policy expert and will provide some context for the story and dialogue that follows. In this case, David Morris is a long-time scholar of the problem of pain who was also involved in the earliest discussions of the idea for this collection.

The bulk of each book will then be devoted to a short but rich narrative written by a patient who has a particular illness or medical problem. As is the case in this particular book, the patient may have found the medical system wanting in approach, behavior, and even philosophy. Finally, a concluding section will be written by a clinician involved in the care of this particular problem or group of patients. The purpose of this clinical commentary is not to enter into a debate or argument with the patient. The doctor or other clinician will not try to argue the patient out of his or her feelings and beliefs, dispute the validity of the diagnosis, or question if the patient really was treated as described. Rather, the clinician will use his or her expertise to understand the patient's account and to help others—both patients and clinicians alike—learn from it.

As the initial volume in the collection, this book serves as a template. David Morris, who is all too familiar with patients whose pain has been poorly managed, leads us into this ill-charted terrain in which those who vow to do no harm inadvertently do precisely the opposite. Lous Heshusius, the author, invites us along as she tries to navigate this harrowing journey through the world of pain, where she encounters health professionals of various types who have difficulty providing the kind of guidance and help she so desperately needs. Finally, Scott M. Fishman, a physician who specializes in pain medicine, stands back and reflects on Heshusius's experience and helps us understand, from the clinician's point of view, how things could go so wrong and how we can all learn to right them.

Sometimes the clinical commentator and patient will not agree about the dotting of every i and crossing of every *t*. In this case, for example, they do not entirely agree about the benefits or potential side effects of a therapy that the author found enormously helpful. Nonetheless, the three participants in this journey—and those who will be presented in subsequent volumes—join in their fundamental understanding that clinicians and patients must work not in isolation but together if medicine is to fulfill its promise.

Suzanne Gordon and Sioban Nelson

Foreword

David B. Morris

In a memoir remarkable for its rare combination of intimate self-revelation and careful research, Lous Heshusius recalls a moment that brings her face-to-face with the unexpected consequences and unanswerable questions that typify chronic pain. Suddenly, gazing at a photo that shows her prior to the automobile accident that damaged her neck, she grasps the transformation that has utterly shattered both her life and her identity. "I had become someone else," she writes. "'A crumbled woman,' is how one of my daughters described me. A strange shadow of my former self. Yet, I have an intimate knowledge of this person in the picture. I know how she thought, felt, loved, walked, and worked. The kind of mother she was. I know the shades of her emotions. I understand how her mind worked. I like this woman. I want to be her. How did she slip through my fingers?"

"Crumbled" is the word she also uses to describe the twisted steel beams of the wrecked car that precipitated her injury. She too is wrecked. Her closing question—less an inquiry than a lament—highlights more than the experience of loss so central to the experience of chronic pain patients. It also points toward larger questions implicitly raised by the new series on how patients think that her book initiates.

As the series editors point out, two books with the title *How Doctors Think* describe the myths and realities of clinical judgment. As Dr. Scott Fishman writes in a clinical commentary that follows Heshusius's narrative, physicians are always constrained by their need to calculate (on behalf of the patient) a balance between risk and benefit.[1] Doctors also calculate the risk-benefit balance, as Fishman explains, for doctors themselves. "Calculation" may be the key term here. Patients, as Lous Heshusius helps us recognize, think differently. Which is why this book, difficult as it may be for doctors, nurses, social workers (as well as for patients and family members) is such an important addition to the literature of patient narratives. At times angry, and certainly sorrowful, her narrative can help us navigate the pain that so often comes with the sudden shock of an unimaginable, total disruption of our everyday lives and purposes.

The scene in which Lous Heshusius examines an old photo—comparing the wrecked patient with her healthy alter ego—holds iconic power to evoke some of the distinctive qualities that mark patients' thinking. It is thinking in which far more goes on than the exercise of judgment and the calculation of risks and benefits. It is a thinking in which feeling, intuition, and memory play a more important role than the instrumental reason basic to scientific research and to clinical medicine. As patients cross the chasm that divides a healthy past from a pain-filled present, memory does not involve the accurate recall of information, which computers perform flawlessly and unfeelingly, but an imperfect, uncontrolled upwelling of what the distinguished chemist and philosopher Michael Polanyi called "personal knowledge."[2] It is a way of thinking, unlike clinical medicine based on best practices, that must push beyond what is objectively or measurably knowable: *I know the shades of her emotions. I understand how her mind worked. I like this woman."*

Doctors don't usually think this way both because they can't afford to (given the current market model of medicine) and because they are trained not to. They may eventually, however, come to see both medical and economic value in recognizing how patients think. Empathy—highly valued in medical education today—would seem impossible without an effort to understand the distinctive patterns of patients' thinking. The way patients think clearly affects behaviors relevant to medical care. It affects compliance. It affects return visits and doctor-shopping. It affects the possibilities of healing.

How we think, in short, is as important as what we think *about,* and thinking may have as many variants as pain. Just as cancer pain differs from neuropathic pain, low back pain, or the pain of migraine, thinking includes significantly different styles. Martin Heidegger's *What Is Called Thinking?* (1954) devotes its entire first half to an extended reflection on a single sentence from the pre-Socratic philosopher Parmenides. For Heidegger, rigorous philosophical thinking clearly differs from the ordinary process later described by neuroscientist Antonio Damasio that involves reason in complex cortical networks connected to memory and emotion.[3] Doctors, in effect, need to unlearn ordinary thought in order to pursue a calculating, logic-based, evidence-based, analytical, objective, risk-benefit thinking in which reason is an instrument for achieving clinical results. Patients, by contrast, embrace a far less instrumental style of reasoning. Joan Didion, in *The Year of Magical Thinking* (2000), describes how her bereavement included a "disordered" thought process not simply emotional but almost mythic in its power to remake actuality.[4] Lous Heshusius shows how pain puts into play not only personal knowledge and emotional intelligence but also nonconscious mental actions ranging from habit to dreamwork.

Pain may have an uncanny power to throw us back on thinking styles absolutely basic to who we are—and we are all different. Differences in ethnicity and in culture affect the experience of pain. Patients from minority groups—African Americans and Latinos, for example—often receive less emergency room medication for pain than do white patients, just as minorities in poor neighborhoods have more limited access to pain-relieving drugs. Lous Heshusius is thrown back on the thinking basic to her life as an academic. Pain sets her a problem that she tackles with the skills of a researcher or project manager in search of specialized expertise: "There have been some 240 appointments with doctors and specialists, and nearly 500 appointments with alternative professionals to date. Add to that about a dozen appointments for tests and assessments....I also attended a ten-day residential pain clinic. I have seen my prolotherapist in Vancouver thirteen times so far, a full day of travel each time. Add countless hours have been spent making lists of questions for all these professionals, keeping track of prescriptions, bills, insurance correspondence, learning about chronic pain...all this on top of 'managing' thousands of hours of pain."

How far is the experience described by Lous Heshusius *representative?* Scott Fishman sees her dilemma within the health-care system as all too common. Still, generalizations about pain patients or about chronic pain need adjustment for real-world variants. Some people in pain are thrown back on thinking styles more closely connected with churches and spiritual practices than with universities. Others, skeptical of all professions, clergy and doctors alike, refuse to classify themselves as patients or to enter the medical system. Still others have no health insurance and thus no access to the world of pain medicine. These nonpatients may ride out their affliction with native stoicism, resignation, prayer, alcohol, or unrelieved anguish. Because the medical research on pain draws almost entirely on patient populations for its statistical findings, we know very little about how nonpatients deal with chronic pain. Anecdotal evidence suggests that some people in chronic pain (remaining outside the medical systems that define them as patients) invent personalized coping styles that permit them to achieve, by their own accounts, successful and happy lives.

There is growing medical literature on "pain beliefs." The beliefs that patients hold, knowingly or unknowingly, alter both pain intensity and pain-related quality of life. Beliefs about pain, for example, have more influence on quality of life than does pain intensity. Moreover, pain patients function better when they believe in their own self-efficacy, believe that they have some control over their pain, and believe that they are not severely disabled.[5] Some pain beliefs can cause direct harm, and among the most harmful pain beliefs for patients is the cognitive-emotional state known as *catastrophizing,* or "characterizations of pain as awful, horrible and unbearable."[6]

I want to be absolutely clear that I cannot and do not offer any medical judgment about Lous Heshusius. Her narrative, however, describes experience that surely resembles a *catastrophe* in the original Greek sense (meaning, "an overturning, a sudden turn"). The nightmares that she narrates so vividly reflect a life in which daylight thinking, like nighttime dreaming, regularly encounters incomprehension and terror. For some people, chronic pain is in fact an abrupt descent into prolonged disaster. "In this book I show as clearly as I can," Heshusius writes soberly, "what happens when a life that is going along just fine takes that sudden turn into the hell that is chronic pain."

The underworld journey—a classic narrative motif—operates for Heshusius less as an ordering structure than as a submerged metaphor that on occasion rises into plain sight. It is important, however, to recognize that what she gives us with her journal-based realism must necessarily take the written form of a narrative, and narratives (never merely an objective record of facts and events) offer revelations both direct and indirect. Doctors are now taking a serious look at the possibilities of a narrative medicine, as narrative not only provides a unique access to patient experience but also reveals how, in less obvious ways, individual and cultural stories help *to shape* the individual experience of illness.[7] For example, there is both narrative knowledge and medical value in the recognition that, at moments, dying to Lous Heshusius seems like welcome freedom: "Death appears kind to me, not like pain, whom I imagine as a devil with raked horns." Attention to narrative would reveal that even the act of narration at times, for Lous Heshusius, resembles a mortal combat between good and evil: "Another reason to write this book has been to get even with Pain. When I find the words that come close to grasping the reality of living with severe chronic pain, I rise to Pain's devilish power."

An established religious vocabulary linking pain with Satan, sin, and death reflects various traditions that view pain as an unmitigated evil. What matters here is both its relevance to the experience of a postmodern academic woman with nontraditional religious views as well as its contribution to her gathering narrative about a contemporary underworld journey. It is, as Dr. Fishman observes, also a journey through a health-care system that for many patients is itself "a major source of both pain and suffering." With Lous Heshusius as a guide, pain patients can learn much here about the perils of a modern health-care odyssey. Health professionals can learn how an articulate middle-class female white patient *thinks* (with all that thinking entails) when her world is irreversibly altered by pain. She does not promise happy endings. Chronic pain is like that. We do not know (such is the honest power of her narrative) if Lous Heshusius will ever fully emerge, like Dante from a different inferno, into the light. From the rare intersection in this text between patient narrative and physician response, however, readers may construct a dialogue on pain in our time that cannot fail to bring plentiful opportunities for personal insight and professional enlightenment.

Acknowledgments

During the years this book was slowly emerging, a number of people were significantly involved in my life and thus in the making of the book. In the world of medicine, I am deeply indebted to Dr. Nasif Yasin, specialist in Rehabilitation and Physical Medicine in Vancouver, for giving me a life back with his skillful prolotherapy treatments. His humanity and skill will always be with me. I thank Dr. Gordon Ko, director of the Canadian Centre for Integrative Medicine in Toronto, and Dr. Stan Gerhart and Dr. Charles Meyers for their compassionate care and open-minded approaches to dealing with my pain problems. My deepest gratitude goes to psychotherapist Brian Grady, the most vigilant listener I have ever known, always ready to hear the misery I bring while grounding me back into life. I thank Lynn Smith for being a most compassionate and excellent masseuse. Thanks also to the staff at the Royal Jubilee Hospital Pain Clinic in Victoria, in particular staff member Linda Cundiff, for the patient-oriented atmosphere they create.

For encouraging reactions to earlier drafts or to parts of the manuscript, I would like to acknowledge Gerry Daly, Merry Connor, Leah Fowler, Maxine Demmler, Alan Cassels, and Arild Solbakken. For their in-depth reading and extensive feedback I gratefully acknowledge Dr. Annette Grundholm, my daughter Renee Gilsdorf, and professor of Pediatrics at Brown Medical School, in Providence, Rhode Island, Bonnie O'Connor. Their comments made me rethink some insights and sharpen others. I was also fortunate that Robert Amussen agreed to carefully read the manuscript. His marvelous editing skills and sensitivity to my experiences made reviewing his comments not a task but a great pleasure.

Very special thanks to James Henry, scientific director of the Michael G. DeGroote Institute for Pain Research and Care at McMaster University in Hamilton, Ontario. I, a stranger, dared to send him my manuscript. His enthusiastic response and recognition of the importance of knowledge gained from real life brought welcome encouragement and validation. I also thank him and sociology professor Arthur Frank of the University of Calgary for establishing contact with Cornell University Press on my behalf.

My many thanks to co-editors of this series Suzanne Gordon and Sioban Nelson for their immediate enthusiasm for this work and for suggestions on restructuring certain aspects of the manuscript. It was Suzanne Gordon's idea to ask David Morris, professor in both the Department of English and the Center for Bioethics and Humanities at the University of Virginia, and Dr. Scott Fishman, chief of Pain Medicine at the University of California at Davis, for their commentary. And while one could not expect full agreement between the way people living with the complexity of chronic pain see their lives and a professional's understanding of it, Dr. Fishman and professor Morris come as close as one could hope. Their own writings on pain have been important in the shaping of my work, and it is an honor to see their words next to mine.

For their assistance in manuscript preparation I thank editorial director of ILR Press Frances Benson and her kind and helpful staff at Cornell University Press. I appreciate the fine editorial work by Ange Romeo-Hall, senior manuscript editor, and by Katy Meigs, copyeditor. Many thanks also to Andy Stewart for gently and cheerfully dealing with my self-created program-formatting headaches.

I am profoundly grateful to Michael Wheeler and Gerry Daly who were there to help when I needed it during the most terrible years in Toronto. For their support and friendship I further thank Maxine Demmler, Norah Harris, Leah Fowler, and Robert Arril, and for their support from afar my sister Ton Waagmeester, Linda Ware, Michiel Kolman, Loree Rackstraw, and Leslie Broun.

I am grateful to fellow pain sufferers, Liesl Fulton, Annette Goranson, and Carol Baddeley for validating so much of my experiences by sharing theirs, and for the solace that brings. I love my cats, Chester, Liefke, Milton, and Hombre for their unwavering daily companionship. I could not live my pained days without them. I also wish to acknowledge political satirists Jon Stewart and Stephen Colbert: their sanity somehow helps me to keep mine.

To my daughters, Nicolle and Renee, I can only say: Thank you for being there. Without you I would no longer be here. Your support and love through these years has been vital to my survival.

I dedicate this book to all sentient beings in pain—whether unavoidable, undertreated, ignored, or inflicted.

Introduction

How do you put hell on paper? Love would be easier. Or joy, or pleasure. Things people desire. Then you can evoke that which cannot be said. The reader will gladly fill in the meanings left unsaid by words. Trying to speak of chronic pain, on the other hand, the unsaid meanings are not easily imagined. For who wants to know what constant pain is like? How to tell of this dark, dark place?

Always inadequately. It means searching for ways that tell what is nearly impossible to describe, for pain has no external referent. We cannot point to pain. It is internal, subjective, and undesired, making the telling about it extremely difficult. Why, then, attempt to do what seems unattainable? This book is a lengthy answer to that question, summarized by Elaine Scarry when she says that the act of verbally expressing pain is a necessary prelude to the collective task of diminishing pain.[1]

I read Scarry's words in the midst of working on this book and they struck a nerve. For as the pain persisted, from weeks to months to years, and became chronic and severe, I had come to experience that, indeed, living with chronic pain—though intensely personal—is not a rugged, individual process but involves every aspect of one's life and every person in one's life. Chronic pain involves complex pathways involving body and mind, emotions and the brain, and diminishing it is not often something a doctor can do on her or his own. Instead, diminishing pain is a multifaceted effort that calls for receptivity and engagement on the part of many.

However, the chronic pain experience is so invisible, so undramatic from the outside—we look normal, we are not terminally ill—that it is an illness still largely hidden from view, its nature ill understood except by the sufferer. In this book I show as clearly as I can, what happens when a life that is going along just fine takes that sudden turn into the hell that is chronic pain.

I was born in the Netherlands where I had a very good childhood. I became a teacher and took a teaching job in South America where I met my former husband, who was from the United States. We moved to Illinois and later lived in various places in the United States. We had two daughters. I left the marriage in the mid-1970s and went to graduate school to study special education and educational research methodology. I became a university professor, first at the University of Northern Iowa, and for the last two decades at York University in Toronto, where I greatly enjoyed teaching and doing research.

Life was good—until that inattentive moment when I did not see the car coming. It happened in the countryside, two hours north of Toronto. It was a late September afternoon in 1996. It had just started to rain and darkness was setting in. My small Pontiac Firefly had no chance against the large dark green Buick that hit me at ninety kilometers per hour while I was pulling away from a stop sign. I was unconscious for half an hour and still have no memory of any of it. A matter of momentary inattention. A lapse that altered my life. And possibly the lives of the people in the other car.

The police officer who came to the hospital that night, told me they had found me inside the car and had feared I was dead. It took them twenty minutes to get me out, trapped as I was between the driver's door and the crumbled steel of the passenger seat that was pushed up against me. I had been hit from the passenger's side, my car pushed across the intersection, thrown into the ditch, and turned on its side. The officer questioned me as I lay there, having barely regained consciousness. I asked if he could come back the next day as I was too exhausted. "No," he said, "tomorrow is my day off."

For me, tomorrow turned out to be the beginning of the kind of life I could not have imagined. Since the accident, pain has altered and tormented every aspect of my life. For the first few years I continued to work part time, albeit with great difficulty, taking two sick leaves. Eventually, the pain became so constant and severe that I had no choice but to go on disability leave. In 2002 I moved to Victoria, British Columbia, to be closer to my daughters and to escape the harsh Toronto winters that invariably made living with pain worse. By the time I moved, I had seen over twenty doctors and specialists and had been subjected to an array of medical treatments. Some brought temporary relief. Some made the pain worse. None brought a cure.

From the very beginning of this tormenting journey I scribbled notes on whatever was happening with me. This practice was crucial for my psychological and emotional survival and resulted in hundreds of pages of notes, jotted down initially with no intent to do anything with them. When in 2004 I finally found some relief with prolotherapy, I began to realize that there was enough "data" to organize these notes into a book.[2] Given that too little is known about the day-to-day suffering of those in pain and the impact chronic pain has on a life—and hence, too little attention and too few resources are directed our way—I felt my story needed to see the light of day.

I decided that if I were to engage this difficult task, the only way to proceed would be with total honesty. That means that as my story takes shape there are many moments of despair, bewilderment, and grief, and many moments of feeling abandoned by doctors and friends alike. Often these moments appear as they did in my journals in all their sharpness. I ask the reader to bear with me, as I slowly learn to place these moments in the larger contexts of cultural and human complexities and suffering of all kinds.

On its website, the American Pain Foundation (APF) cites the figure of 75 million people in the United States living with pain, 42 percent of them—roughly 31 million—for longer than one year. Pain, according to the APF, affects more Americans than diabetes, heart disease, and cancer combined. The estimate by the National Institute of Neurological Disorders and Stroke puts the figure of people living with pain at 90 million.[3] The Canadian Pain Coalition estimates the figure for Canada to be almost 6 million.[4] "The problem is absolutely enormous," Russell Portenoy, chair of Pain Medicine at New York's Beth Israel Medical Center, told Steve Sternberg and reported in a *USA TODAY* article on May 8, 2005. He added, "It rivals every serious public-health issue, whether you're talking about heart disease, cancer, obesity or anything else." Yet most people never see the pain in these millions of sufferers, even when they stand next to them on a bus or in the supermarket. And while doctors can see heart disease, cancer, obesity and most other diseases, they, too, cannot see pain.

The problem is also costly. The APF estimates the annual cost in the Unites States of chronic pain, including health-care expenses, lost income, and lost productivity, to be $100 billion. In Canada these costs are estimated to be $45 billion, which includes the cost for long-term disability.[5]

Chronic pain and the problems and questions it generates is no respecter of national boundaries. Most of my story takes place in Toronto and in Victoria, British Columbia. I also attended a pain clinic in Amsterdam and one in the United States near Seattle. The debates about how to diagnose and treat chronic pain are much the same internationally and characterized by much uncertainty and contradictions.

At the Congressional Briefing on Pain on Capitol Hill held June 13, 2006, chronic pain was referred to as the "silent epidemic."[6] It is an invisible epidemic, the severity of which is greatly underestimated because few people know about our lives in any depth. David Morris, in *The Culture of Pain*, captures the lack of knowledge about our lives well: "Chronic pain may push us toward an area of human life we know almost nothing about.... It places people in utterly different worlds of feeling. It surrounds them with silence. In many ways the person in chronic pain might as well be standing on the moon."[7]

Ralph Waldo Emerson said of pain: "He has seen but half the universe who has not been shown the house of pain."[8] I hope my tale will take the reader some way into that house of pain, and in doing so contribute to its eventual lessening.

Inside Chronic Pain

1   *A Life Altered*

The Descent

The emergency room nurse told me I had been in a serious accident about two hours north of Toronto. "You will feel pain in places where you never thought you could have pain," she said. I had no memory of the accident—and still don't. I had visited another land, noticing nothing of police cars and ambulances. I had been to an alternate, beautiful reality. When I came to, I felt myself inside a brilliant light. Opening my eyes, I saw smiling faces of young men against a clear blue sky. The color of the air was of golden sunshine. The world felt wonderful. I felt rested. Not a touch of fatigue. I felt such joy. I was in a space lighter and more beautiful than I had ever known, than I knew was possible. A space I wanted to dwell in forever.

But it rained. It was late September, the afternoon darkening. I was five minutes away from a friend's house when I did not see the car coming. The faces above me belonged to three paramedics who were holding a large umbrella over me. I saw no sky. There was no sun. Just worried faces looking at me. I was on a stretcher. They were getting ready to put me in the ambulance. I learned later that had my bones not been so strong, as indicated by bone density tests, my neck would have been broken. I might have gone to that other side forever. Often, in the terror caused by the pain that followed, I have wished for that. Such a painless journey it would have been. Straight to paradise.

When the nurse said those words, I remember thinking: "Oh, you don't know how healthy I am. I'm never sick! I'll recover from this in no time!" But she was right. What she didn't tell me, however, was that I would see numerous doctors and specialists and that still my pain would continue. Now, after more than eleven years, three family doctors, two neurospecialists, four pain specialists, two neurological surgeons, a psychiatrist, an anesthesiologist, a neuropsychiatrist, an osteopathic physician, three chiropractors, a holistic physician, a wellness physician, two acupuncturists, two physiotherapy programs, three individual physiotherapists, one emotional release therapist, a marijuana specialist, a pain/trauma therapist, two psychotherapists, a cognitive therapist, two osteopaths, a biofeedback therapist, two craniosacral therapists, ten days in a private residential pain clinic, about a dozen massage therapists, uncounted painkillers, and a losing fight with the insurance company, I continue to suffer daily from stabbing neck and head pain, from migraines, from referred pain throughout my left shoulder and upper back, and from neuropathic pain that causes swelling in my neck and at the back of my skull and that causes a stinging and burning sensation.

As time went on, I came to understand that the words "chronic pain" essentially mean "You have had pain now for over half a year and we have no real clue what to do about it." Then, guided by the war-and-control metaphors of much conventional medicine, many drugs are prescribed, toxic substances injected, and burn-or-cut-the-nerves procedures carried out, none of which offer certainty, all of which carry risks. There was no one to help me sort out the piecemeal and contradictory information doctors and specialists would provide, nearly all of which was new to me. One pain specialist did his best, but his full waiting room and his fast mind—way too fast for me—did not often allow for a coherent explanation in the short time he had available.

I used to divide my life into "Before" and "After": before and after I had children; before and after I left my marriage; before and after the love of my life appeared and had to part. Clearly, these continue to be significant milestones in my life. But nothing has divided in two the before and after of my life as did the accident that left me a victim of the chronic pain that has tormented me ever since. Albert Schweitzer said, "We all must die. But if I can save him from days of torture, that is what I feel is my great and ever new privilege. Pain is a more terrible lord of mankind than even death himself."[1]

Death. How often have I wished I could lie down and simply die. I can put it in writing: had it not been for my two daughters, I would no longer be here. A Google search on the relation between chronic pain and suicide brings up almost a million hits. Many articles note a significantly higher rate of suicide ideation and suicide attempts among those living with chronic pain than for the general population. The Johns Hopkins Arthritis Center reports a two to three times higher rate of actual suicides for chronic pain patients than for the general population.[2] In his review of research dealing with the impact of chronic pain on life habits, James Henry, scientific director of the Michael G. DeGroote Institute for Pain Research and Care at McMaster University, cites reports that among medical illnesses, chronic pain is the second major cause of suicide after bipolar disorder, and ahead of depression and psychotic disorders.[3]

Ongoing intense pain then is for many chronic pain sufferers worse than the idea of death. Yet no one responded when I expressed suicidal thoughts, which during the worst years were present on a daily basis and about which, out of absolute despair, I tried to talk with six health-care professionals. "Let's not go there," was the immediate response from one of them. The others simply said nothing. Tellingly, however, it did show up in some of the reports they wrote to each other.

Many times I have promised God, who I had set aside some forty years ago for the notion of Spirit or Creative Force, that I will never complain about anything anymore if He or She would relieve me from this pain. Many times I have moaned and whispered, "Please, let it pass!" with the strong sense I was directing my prayer to something more personal than a spirit or a force. "*Ik kan het niet meer,*" I moaned, falling back into Dutch, my native tongue. "I can't go on anymore." Though I left the Netherlands over forty years ago, my mother tongue still rises up in me in moments of great intensity or great despair.

Why I Write This Book: Witnessing Lives in Pain

Carol Jay Levy in *A Pained Life,* her account of her struggle with pain from trigeminal neuralgia, gives as the reason for not writing her story sooner that the story would not have had a happy ending.[4] When at last a neurological implant took her pain away she could write because her story now had a happy ending. How we want happy endings. In *The*

Wounded Storyteller Arthur Frank refers to stories that tell about restoring the former state of health as "restitution narratives," which, he says, are the ones that get attention.[5] But the world also needs to witness the stories of pain that go on with no end in sight. Those where health is not restored. Those that end in despair. In death. How else can the torment of chronic pain be understood, rather than greatly underestimated, as I now know it is? The entire range of pain stories needs to be acknowledged to encourage political and social progress on the pain-management front.

It is difficult to imagine a life in chronic pain. Apart from being invisible and inexpressible, the intensity, frequency, and duration of pain attacks differ for everyone and can change over time. NBC's *The Today Show* aired a series on chronic pain beginning on March 28, 2005. It noted six defining characteristics: (1) when it interferes with activity, (2) when it interferes with concentration, (3) when it disrupts sleep, (4) when one self-medicates, (5) when it strains relationships, and (6) when it appears regularly—meaning three times a month or more. These defining characteristics, while offering an initial screen, are so broad that they do not provide a means to diagnose the severity of the pain or to imagine what a life in pain is like. The ubiquitous 1–10 pain scale does not do so either.

I once attended a demonstration organized by a company that designs products for pain relief. Before the demonstration began, the presenter asked, "How many of you, right now, have a pain level of 10 on a scale from 1 to 10, in which 10 is the worst pain you can imagine?" About a dozen people raised their hands. They had been walking around, chatting, and having refreshments before the demonstration started. I was stunned. At a 10 I am on the floor, motionless, with gunshots going off in my head. Some months later I am in my specialist's office for injections. I can hear every word said by the patient behind the curtain on the cot next to mine. The specialist asks, "What's your pain level today on a scale of 1 to 10?"

"About a 10." I am stunned again. At a 10 level of pain I could not have possibly come to the clinic. When my turn comes I tell him what I overheard. "At a 10 I am motionless on the floor." He explains that the scale—used only for intrapersonal comparison—has no comparative value. One person's level 6 bears no necessary comparison to another person's level 6. A 2007 special issue on chronic pain by *Newsweek* calls this scale—so far, according to the magazine, the best that clinicians have been able to come up with—"absurdly imprecise."[6]

If the goal is to be precise, it must be said that the pain scale is imprecise even for intrapersonal comparisons. Every time I have to indicate where my pain is on this scale, I hesitate. Typically, the pain patient is asked to mark the scale according to how the pain is "Now" or "Today." There is of course a distinct difference between a 2 and a 9, or between a 3 and 8. But the shorter the distances between numbers, the more the meanings of these distances start to blur. After eleven years of this, I still don't know what, exactly, the difference between a 6 and a 7 is or between a 6 and an 8. Nor what a 3 really means. Or a 4. Just as important, the doctor has no idea. There is nothing to back up the number. Therefore, a 5 is not always a 5. It depends on my day. The pain's fluctuations—often within minutes or within hours—blur these numbers. My mood of the day blurs these numbers. Whether or not I have taken painkillers blurs these numbers. My inexact memory of what the pain was like last time I marked the scale a certain way—which, in order for the scale to be valid, one would need to assume I can remember—blurs these numbers. The way a particular doctor behaves toward me blurs these numbers.

Fluctuations in chronic pain are typical. I never make morning appointments, because the pain is typically too severe for me to go anywhere. Thus my afternoon marks are a serious understatement of the severity of the pain I live with. I tell doctors about the morning pain, but we largely believe only what we can see, and doctors are not exempt from this human tendency—in fact, their scientific training reinforces it. A physician who read the manuscript for this book told me, "I will never again say to myself when listening to a patient talking about pain, 'It can't be that bad—she seems pretty normal to me.'"

One of my pain specialists told me of his frustration over how to define chronic pain to an insurance representative. He finally said, "Imagine someone stabbing you in the back, not once, not twice, but many times a day, day after day, month after month, year after year, and you don't know why he is stabbing you." He shook his head as he told me this.

I tried to explain chronic pain to an acquaintance who couldn't understand why I couldn't teach anymore or take a trip, and why I couldn't just take some pain killers and wouldn't that get rid of the pain? Trying to come up with a picture that would make the invisible visible, I heard myself say, "Imagine you wake up every morning and you need to go to a clinic down the road for painful treatments that take a couple of hours and for which only a mild anesthetic can be given. You have to do that every day, at least once, sometimes more often—for years on end. Possibly for the rest of your life." "Oh…" he said, falling silent, struggling to get that image into his head. Coming up with concrete images that resemble what the chronic pain experience is like may be crucial in the struggle to give voice to this insidious disease that few understand and many don't even believe is real.

Another way to show what living chronically in pain is like is to register the frequency and intensity of the pain and the consequences for daily life. Using various pain diaries I kept for medical and legal reasons during the worst years and estimating the number of hours for the subsequent years, I can roughly calculate the number of hours I have suffered from pain. However, these hours are not all the same when it comes to pain intensity. The literature on pain rarely distinguishes between levels of pain or systematically indicates their different consequences. For me, the following three levels of pain have been almost separate illnesses each with its own set of consequences.

Severe pain (for me, I would mark between an 8 and 10 rating on the scale) means to me pain so intense that it completely disables. Pain that paralyzes. Pain that erases the mind and can make you irrational. Pain that makes it impossible to work, to drive, to converse, to sleep. Pain that is hardly responsive to medication. The kind of pain that makes you suicidal. That kind of pain lives off the scale, somewhere between 11 and infinity. For then, *all* of me is pain. It is an altered state in which the notion of ranking is no longer valid. To call total pain a 10, or any number at all, feels strange—a number only makes sense if there is another number to compare it with. When pain is total, there is no entity with which to compare it.

Considerable pain (a 5–7 rating) to me is pain that, with dulling medication, allows one to go through the necessary daily activities at home, though not much more. It is pain that does not allow you to work at your job. Pain that makes it dangerous to drive and severely restricts your social life. Pain that exhausts and demands constant attention.

Light pain (a 1–4 rating) is pain that nags, that interferes with clear thinking, with work, with enjoying company. It is pain that responds better to medication and allows for normal home and work activities to go on, but pain that nevertheless brings fatigue, distracts, and makes you less effective at whatever you are doing.

Taken together, I experienced approximately 8,700 hours of severe pain, 7,200 hours of considerable pain, and 11,500 hours of light pain. In all, over 27,000 hours of pain over an eleven-year period. This means an average of approximately seven hours of pain each day, every day. Immediately following the accident there were hours, and sometimes days, with little or no pain. Since my improvement after prolotherapy, there is still pain every day but of less intensity and duration. During the worst four years, however, there was pain all day and all night. Can anyone, not knowing chronic pain, imagine 27,000 hours of pain? The picture is worse, in fact. For these thousands of hours of pain are not predictable as to when they will decide to show up. Therefore, every hour is an hour with pain either present or hovering around. Life becomes pain. *I* become pain. A number on a scale cannot be a witness to this.

Newsweek's observation that the pain scale is "absurdly imprecise," which seems to imply there should be a more precise scale, is not that precise itself. Given pain's invisibility and subjectivity, the notion of "precise" is besides the point: it is not within the realm of the possible. To come up with a 1–10 scale to "measure" pain fits the values of the scientific paradigm in which knowledge is seen to demand measurement in order to be considered valid and reliable. Within this paradigm, to measure means to quantify—to assign numbers to things and to relations between things. This demands counting. But what is there to count?

Here is more or less what goes through my mind when the scale is put in front of me for the umpteenth time: Here we go again. What to mark. Last time I think I said my pain was a 6. But I don't exactly remember how bad the pain was when I circled a 6. Or, I think: I feel only light pain right now. Perhaps I feel a 3. But five minutes from now it may be a 2 or a 4. Becoming impatient with the scale and with my inability to get it "right"—because getting it right is impossible—I just circle a 3. Done. I give the whole thing back to the secretary.

For myself, given I experience three distinct levels of pain, with distinctly different concrete consequences for the *reality* of my day-to-day life, a 1–3 scale—if we have to have a scale—would be more accurate and reliable as an indicator of the severity of pain I live with, particularly if the numbers are accompanied with descriptors of these actual consequences. Some form of a scale combining numbers and consequences might be more helpful for both diagnosis and treatment suggestions and evaluations. It would also help doctors understand the chronic pain experience better, which a number on a scale by itself cannot do. Something meaningful needs to back up the numbers. Since nothing can be actually "counted" or "measured" in today's science, the acts of counting and measuring need to embody something that is directly relevant to lives lived in pain.[7]

There are many books and articles about chronic pain written by medical practitioners. They have been very helpful in giving me some understanding of what was happening to me at the physical level. However, they give the reader little knowledge of what thousands of hours of pain do to a life. There is rarely a sense of the ecology of the pain experience. They are not written to portray how profoundly interactions and relations with others change: with family, friends, colleagues, and even with strangers. Or to provide a clear picture of how one's sense of self is altered, if not destroyed. The social and cultural influences on chronic pain are not often mentioned. This is also the case for self-help books, where chronic pain is mostly presented as an individual and medical problem.

It is much more than that.

Arthur Rosenfeld, a journalist, has captured personal experience through interviews with people living in pain in *The Truth about Chronic Pain*. Rosenfeld also interviewed doctors, theorists, and philosophers.[8] Still, the interviews are structured by Rosenfeld's questions, and the stories gained from them are only a few pages long. Rosenfeld, who does not suffer from chronic pain himself, was bothered, as I am, by the absence in the literature of the voices of those who know chronic pain firsthand. Marni Jackson, also a journalist and the author of *Pain: The Science and Culture of Why We Hurt* and who suffers from migraines herself, offers a very informative narrative constructed from her many interactions with people living with chronic pain, their doctors, and others in the field of pain management.[9] In all, however, little that conveys the depth and detail of day-to-day living in pain, as experienced and recounted by the sufferer, is available.

There are reasons for this. Constant pain steals time and energy by the tons, grabs all one's attention, deadens motivation, robs one of sleep, and brings on depression. In addition, chronic pain is invisible and defeats the power of language to capture it. In David Morris's words, "The normal failure of language under the assault of acute pain…is a common but not devastating experience. A pain that lasts for months or years, however… constitutes a radical assault on language and on human communication."[10] Morris further points out that the Melzack's McGill Pain Questionnaire, used by many doctors, reduces the patient's experience to a mere seventy-eight words that attempt to describe how the physical pain feels. They are useful only to doctors. He adds that "chronic pain opens up an unsocial, wordless terrain where all communication threatens to come to a halt….Its inarticulate silences serve as the expression of an otherness so alien that we have no words and no language with which to comprehend it."

His words tighten my chest. I know them to be true. Morris stresses, as I do, the immense difference between acute pain and chronic pain, which goes on for years. While acute pain gets wide attention, those living with chronic pain soon discover, as Morris notes, that their complaints—potentially endless—often exhaust, frustrate, and finally alienate family, friends, and physicians. As a result, they learn to keep it to themselves. After eleven years of suffering from chronic pain, I know he is right. How, then, could I even imagine writing a book about this devastating experience not many want to hear about—an experience for which there is no proper language?

It has been an act of instinct and survival. This book grew out of years of making notes, a stream of pained, fractured consciousness, scribbled at first instinctively, only to serve as a witness to my own altered life. As time passed, however, and I learned how others, including many health-care professionals, fail to grasp the torment that is chronic pain, I needed to try to be a witness for the larger world as well. My scribbles offered themselves as the raw data from which I constructed this book. Without them there would be no book. My memory would not have been able to trace the traumas nor the details of events. My psyche would have repressed most of it.

In 2000 the U.S. Congress declared the first decade of this century the "Decade of Pain Control and Research." My experience convinces me that pain control and research *must* systematically incorporate the personal, social, and spiritual aspects of what it's like to live with chronic pain as understood by those living it. If not, pain management will stay within the confines of pharmaceutical and surgical interventions that for many of us are clearly inadequate.

Many of the medical texts on chronic pain use war-and-control metaphors—they are about "waging war" on pain, "conquering" pain, the "battle" with pain, "getting a grasp" on your pain. And while the pieces of my life that fell around me, shattering the very sense of "me," did resemble a battlefield for so many years, I knew that if I were to stay alive, the path ahead of me could not be warlike. Instead, I have had to desperately search for meaning, for a purpose, and for sources of peace. I came to realize how important it is for everyone suffering from this devastating illness to find *something* that transcends the reign of pain, to engage something truly purposeful to which the mind and the emotions still want to go.

Initially, my scribbles served such a purpose. Mostly, I wrote or typed wildly, short statement after short statement, as the pain could not bear to think itself into longer thoughts. These scribbles gave me both an intimate "other" to go to and a place to keep emotions, thoughts, and experiences from being lost. My scribbles are there. They cannot run away, as have friends and colleagues, as well as many doctors. They are waiting for me.

This was particularly important during the worst four years, from mid-1999, when the pain had become intense and constant and the health-care profession showed itself helpless, to the end of 2003, when prolotherapy slowly began to diminish both the intensity and frequency of the pain. During these four years, death wishes predominated in my thoughts, for madness seemed right around the corner. Madness *is* right around the corner when you are in constant severe pain. You are so alone in the pain experience, and there are so few words that can convincingly describe the pain to anyone that you begin to feel that nothing outside the self can be grasped anymore. That nothing is there in any reliable manner. Even thoughts disappear in the agony of pain and of diminished concentration and memory function. As the pain acquires a will of its own, as your relations with the outside world fall apart and friends fall silent, as clerks at the supermarket checkout ask cheerfully, "How are you today?" and you lie, as one doctor says one thing and the other says something quite different, all reliable notions in your world dissolve. You don't even know what your body, your mind, and your emotions will do the next moment. As Dr. Eric Cassell notes in *The Nature of Suffering,* the body in pain is so untrustworthy that it does not even behave consistently.[11] But the scribbles were there to go back to, along with my cats, my music, and the woods outside my window.

I write this book, then, as a witness to lives lived in chronic pain. I want to talk to doctors and connect with pain patients and their families. Some of the things said to me by doctors have been astonishing in a negative way and will find their way into my story. For other doctors, I gained an enormous respect. I told Dr. Gordon Ko, director of the Canadian Centre for Integrative Medicine, the pain clinic I attended in Toronto, that I have no clue how he does it day in, day out with folks like me. He never failed to make me feel better, even when he had to poke needles into me, even when I left his office in tears from pain. He understood. He was kind. Though his waiting room was often full, I always felt he would do anything to find ways to help me. And I will never forget what he said at the end of my first visit, when he called me back as I was walking out of his door: "One more thing, Lous—never give up."

I was taken aback. What was that? Wasn't he supposed to be the one to make me better? At that time I was still under the illusion that chronic pain was a particular kind of pain and that "pain management" clinics were clinics where they knew how to cure you. But he knew better, of course. He was indirectly acknowledging the inability of the medical profession to deal effectively with chronic pain. He was telling me to take charge.

And taking charge is what I ended up having to do, once I realized how uneven knowledge about chronic pain is among physicians and how much disagreement there can be about both diagnosis and treatment. For instance, had I believed the first neurological specialist I saw, I would no longer be able to move my head without being in excruciating pain. Had I believed one anesthesiologist, I would be on daily morphine indefinitely. Had I believed another pain specialist, my only hope would have been the drug Rivotril (the chemical clonazepam) or the use of a transcutaneous electrical nerve stimulation device (TENS), which can inhibit or block the sensation of pain, but which did not work for me. Had I believed still another one, I would have had my nerves burned each year, risking increased pain and the generation of nerve pain. Had I believed one neurosurgeon, I would have had major open neck surgery, with no guarantees and which could have left me with nerve pain that would have never gone away—possible adverse effects he did not even mention.

Then one of my pain specialists in Toronto mentioned prolotherapy in passing, but he took no further action. I did not know what it was and he did not explain. A few weeks before I moved to Victoria, I came upon Dr. Ross Hauser's book *Prolo Your Pain Away!*[12] Reading it, I saw myself described on every page. I read how ligaments that are overstretched and weakened, often by accidents, bring about abnormal motion in the skeletal system, allowing excessive pull on nonstretchable ligament nerve endings, causing local pain as well as referring pain elsewhere in specific and predictable pain patterns. When I read the phrase "a chronically loose joint," I suddenly understood the nature of the strange, shifting feeling inside my neck when I reached out for something, and why the pain would flare up when I did so. I finally understood why I couldn't keep my head up for any length of time and had to lie down many times a day to let it rest. The description of muscle spasms as a result of muscles trying to take over the work of weak, nonfunctional ligaments, explained the constant spasms in my neck and shoulders that caused intense pain.

When I told my pain specialist I was moving to Victoria, he made me promise to see a colleague of his in Vancouver, Dr. Nasif Yasin, a specialist in physical medicine and rehabilitation. As luck would have it, one of the treatments Dr. Yasin specializes in is prolotherapy. I had my first treatment in July 2003. So far, prolotherapy has not cured me, and I continue to "qualify" as a chronic pain patient. I still suffer from considerable pain that wakes me after only a few hours of sleep, pain that often still takes hours to settle. But prolotherapy has reduced both the intensity, frequency, and duration of the pain and has greatly increased the stability and range of motion of my neck. Most afternoons and evenings are now functional as long as I carefully monitor everything I do.

Of course I recognize that what has worked for me may not work for others and that treatments that have helped others may not help me. The same holds for medications. There are no guarantees. This is the nature of chronic pain. Each person reacts individually. But I had to learn that. For the first few years I thought that there was going to be a miracle treatment, somewhere, offered by someone. Instead, it turned out that finding relief is a matter of trial and error, and that many of us need various approaches to pain reduction at the same time. In writing my story then, I am not touting any particular medical approach. I am just recording my story. But it is a story that illustrates the often relentless journey that pain patients have to travel in their search for relief, who meets them, and how they are dealt with along the way. It tells of the patience that is demanded by doctors and patients alike and of the need to broaden the base of possible treatments. The essential message is that giving up—by doctors or by patients—is not an option. Or shouldn't be. If one approach does not work, others need to be explored.

Another reason to write this book has been to get even with Pain. When I find the words that come close to grasping the reality of living with severe chronic pain, I rise to Pain's devilish power. We are on a level playing field. "You need to do what you need to do," I tell it. "But I will do what I need to do." I want Pain to know that it cannot prevent me from making meaning out of its invading my life, from telling the world about its torturous deeds.

Then, I will find moments of happiness, of beauty, of insight—moments few and far between in those thousands of hours of pain. I still find it hard to believe such moments did exist even during the worst years. But they did and I will try to capture them as well.

2   *That Which Has No Words,*
That Which Cannot Be Seen

The Invisible and the Inexpressible

The most pervasive problem of the chronic pain experience, apart from the torment of the pain itself, is its inexpressibility and its invisibility. Much of my story must be understood in the light of this difficulty.

Researcher David Morris tells of his reaction when first talking to chronic pain patients: "What surprised me most…was the apparent normal faces of the patients. I had steeled myself to expect agonized expressions and frightful cries."[1] Indeed, we appear normal. That is our liability. One can wince and moan only for so long. There comes a point where giving expression to one's pain takes energy one no longer has. One becomes quiet and pain becomes internalized.

Also, wincing and moaning when in acute pain are instinctive behaviors to which others respond with sympathy. When it becomes clear the pain will not go away, others may feel helpless. They may start to think you are exaggerating. They may be overwhelmed. They change the subject. The person in pain withdraws. You try to keep your composure, to stay coherent, not fall apart. Others will see exhaustion and depression in your face before they see pain.

I cannot count how often I have broken down in tears during the worst years the moment I got into my car after a doctor's appointment. Or after a shopping trip when pain flared up so violently I could hardly get out of the store. Or after a visitor had left and I was alone again. Or the moment my daughters left the house. As the great Greek poet Sappho wrote, "What cannot be said will get wept."[2]

Pain has no external referent, yet it fills you up. You can't point to it, yet it takes over your being. It is expressed by "cries and whispers" as Ingmar Bergman—Sweden's "poet of pain"—showed in his film of the same name in which the identification of pain with death is palpable. When a major pain attack hits, I cannot form words. Thought and language are wiped out. I cannot communicate. When intense pain takes over, nothing else exists. There is only a spot, a point, a sharpened point of nothingness. And yet it is the only spot where one can still *be*. Where there is still life. Life without thoughts. Without emotions. If, when the pain gets really bad, I can stay focused on that spot and stay in it, I can keep from going crazy. It is in that still point that pain stops being pain. And I must stay there. My mind and body motionless. Only focus. For if I waiver, if I think, if I move, if I feel emotions, pain becomes pain again. The difficulty of staying aware during meditation practice pales compared to the single-minded attention required to stay in that point of stillness, of absolute focus, when in great pain. Often I don't manage. I can't stay there. I must return to the devil.

How to write about this? How to bridge the gap between the stabbing inside my neck and skull and the blank page? Constant severe pain lives in silence—it *silences*. I try to tell someone what the pain is like. The words that fall out of my mouth never match what I want to say. What I say sounds like something not worth telling because it is not true. I cannot make it come true in words.

Palliative care physician David Kuhl, author of *What Dying People Want*, says he came to understand that when physical pain is present it is virtually impossible to address psychological and spiritual concerns.[3] When I read Dr. Kuhl's words I felt relief because I had always felt that, somehow, by the sheer force of will, I should be able to address other matters while in great pain. But it is not possible. Serious pain itself *is* an interfering pattern: it floods the brain, which is then no longer available for thought. Simone Weil, the young French philosopher who herself suffered greatly and worked among those who suffered greatly, wrote, "If there is complete absence of physical pain there is no affliction for the soul, because our thoughts can turn to any object...physical pain, and that alone, has the power to chain down our thoughts."[4]

Thoughts and language can only come after the pain has softened. The nineteenth-century French novelist Alphonse Daudet, who suffered from severe pain, wondered, "Are words actually any use to describe what pain...really feels like? Words only come when everything is over, when things have calmed down. They refer only to memory, and are either powerless or untruthful."[5] Pain "drives out language," says Julian Barnes.[6]

No words were ever written while I was in tormenting pain. Some softening had to happen before I could hold a pen or go to the computer. Then, I often added what was happening while scribbling my notes: "I am bursting into tears writing this." Daudet wrote more eloquently, "This note, made quickly, is wooden, inexpressive, solipsistic; but it was written during cruel illness....My anguish is great, I weep as I write."[7] I relate to his need to tell his readers, in essence—do not think that just because I am writing this my pain cannot be that bad. It is.

Elaine Scarry's analysis of the complications of pain's invisibility mirrors my own experience:

> For the person whose pain it is, it is "effortlessly" grasped (that is, even with the most heroic effort it cannot *not* be grasped); while for the person outside the sufferer's body, what is "effortless" is *not* grasping it (it is easy to remain wholly unaware of its existence; even with effort, one may remain in doubt about its existence or may retain the astonishing freedom of denying its existence; and, finally, if with the best effort of sustained attention one successfully apprehends it, the aversiveness of the "it" one apprehends will only be a shadowy fraction of the actual "it").[8]

This difficulty with expression also holds for my medical appointments. I try to speak to doctors about the severity of my pain. My words float strangely in the air. As I pronounce them, I myself become a spectator. As soon as I begin to speak, I am no longer there. Someone else is speaking these words. Someone who has not suffered the pain, for it is so much worse than she says. How can she say so little? How can she be so superficial? In the meantime, I am watching the doctor. Trying to see how he reacts. Did he get it? Should she be more dramatic? More detailed? But how? How can she, how can I, express this prelanguage torment?

Of my many doctors, only three, perhaps four, seemed to grasp what chronic pain does to a life. Perhaps others also did, but they never gave any sign of it. My psychotherapist, who works with many chronic pain sufferers and is the most attentive person I've ever known, follows me as far as any nonsufferer possibly could. The only other person who gives signs of understanding the un-sayability of this pain has been one of my daughters who spends several days at a time with me. "Where are your thoughts going, mum?" she asks with urgency, but knows she cannot follow me where I go. The pain banging, I sink deeper and deeper into a void. She holds on to my arm as if to keep me from falling into it. "I am so afraid" are the only words I can say.

Someone else's pain, then, can never be confirmed and is, therefore, often denied and always underestimated. These truths echo in the stories told by those in chronic pain who speak of doctors, employers, friends, and even family members who think the sufferer is exaggerating, who can't believe it can be all that bad.

This invisible, inexpressible, and misunderstood experience begs for greater public understanding. For myself, as I lost my job, friends, the ability to travel, to plan ahead for as little as a day, my social life gradually disappearing altogether, I had to create a source that would sustain me, an anchor to hold on to. Keeping a journal of events and experiences that were traumatically altering my life became a therapeutic habit. Often I would write daily, sometimes not for days. The entire process was always spontaneous, motivated by the need to render the invisible somewhat visible and to give the inexpressible the most accurate voice possible.

The Uniqueness of Chronic Pain

Chronic pain as contrasted to acute pain is, simply speaking, pain that has decided to hang around. The commonly accepted time period that needs to pass before pain is considered chronic is six months. However, pain physicians Angela Mailis-Gagnon and David Israelson, authors of *Beyond Pain,* believe that after only four weeks, thoughts and emotions, having become entangled with the physical pain, send their own pain signals to the brain, which sets the condition for long-term disability.[9] Dr. Chester Buckenmaier, chief of the U.S. Army Regional Anesthesia and Pain Management

Initiative at Walter Reed Army Medical Center in Washington, DC, locates the very reason for chronic pain in uncontrolled acute pain, effectively erasing the distinction in terms of duration.[10] He sees uncontrolled acute pain as a disease process in itself: the start of chronic pain is *in* uncontrolled acute pain. The Canadian Consortium on Pain Mechanisms Diagnosis and Management describes chronic pain in similar terms: "Acute pain, which was traditionally seen as temporary, is now envisioned as the initiation phase of an extensive, persistent nociceptive and behavioural cascade of reactions triggered by tissue injury. Within minutes of trauma, phenotypic changes are observed in primary afferent [conveying toward the center] and spinal cord nociceptive neurons, and these changes are the basis for long-term sensitization [nociceptive refers to neural processes that process noxious stimuli; phenotypic changes are changes in any observable characteristic or trait of an organism]."[11] Hence, the inadequacy, not to say danger, of the "let's wait and see" approach taken by my doctors at the time of the accident, which typifies the lack of knowledge about chronic pain on the part of many physicians.

A unique aspect of chronic pain lies in others' perception of it. Most people outside the world of medicine connect serious pain to a major disease. But when people know you are not terminally ill, from their perspective, you seem normal. You "just" have pain. That chronic pain is a pathology in itself is not easily grasped by the lay person. As a result, the message often is "It will go away." "You're strong, you'll get over this," a friend told me cheerfully and with great conviction. That was in 1998. "I just know you will beat this. I feel it," said another friend in 2002.

While chronic pain is not an immediate cause of death, in the long run other illnesses develop from the physical, psychological, and emotional stresses. Prolonged pain produces harmful changes in hormonal and metabolic function, including in brain chemicals. It can considerably raise heart rate and blood pressure and weaken the immune system. I myself suffer from constant sleep deprivation, which causes exhaustion and increased sensitivity to pain, cycles of deep depression, and frequent stomach pains, indicating a possible incipient ulcer, a complimentary result of pain, medications, and stress of all these years.

And then there is the unpredictability of chronic pain: when it comes, when it goes, how bad it is, what it allows you to do or not do. You never know. Pain's unpredictability plays havoc with work, family, and social life.

In Marni Jackson's words, "the random power [of pain] to strike makes you feel temporary as a sand castle."[12] In talking to a friend about my pain's unpredictability, I said, "If only I could have pain on Monday, Tuesday, and Wednesday but not the rest of the week, then at least I could work part time. I could plan a trip for the good days." "Oh well," she replied, "no one knows what the next day will bring. We all can have a heart attack tomorrow." Such relativizing comments entirely miss the point. They are "valid" only at the level where it no longer counts: while true in the abstract, they are irrelevant to the day-to-day functioning of living with pain. I often feel my life is nothing but an endless sequence of *pain-recovery-pain-recovery-pain-recovery-pain-recovery*—"recovery" meaning struggling with exhaustion and lack of sleep and trying to stay in the present and somehow giving meaning to the "good" hours. But the cycles—unpredictable in their timing—come too fast.

Contrary to what many people think, one does *not* become inured to constant pain. On the contrary. Pain is always new. Over time the neurological system, being continually aroused, can become so hyperreactive that the slightest thing can trigger the pain mode. Dr. Scott Fishman, chief of Pain Medicine at the University of California at Davis Medical Center and provider of clinical commentary at the end of this book, explains how lasting pain can produce a cycle of chemical and electrical action and reaction that becomes an automatic feedback loop, a chronic, self-perpetuating pain that persists long after the original trauma has healed.[13] Pain, he says, can reconfigure the architecture of the nervous system it invades, changing the very pathways by which pain responses get sent to the brain in such a way as to generate more pain. The immense complication, Dr. Fishman explains, is that when the nervous system is traumatized, we have an insidious case of the enemy having infiltrated the fortress and sabotaging the command center: the pain problem occurs in the same brain that must make sense of it. The nervous system that signals pain as a warning of injury gets stuck in the "on" position. The alarm system is broken and cannot turn itself off. For many of us, this feels like going crazy. Or, as Dr. Fishman states, it's like being fooled by a horrible hallucination.

A person suffering from chronic pain interviewed by Arthur Rosenfeld tells how one of her doctors told her that living with pain was "like diabetes or heart disease, and that lots of people learn to live with those diseases."[14] But, she says, chronic pain is different. It is very different.

3 *Pain and the Self*

This Pain of Mine

When I was reading about chronic pain somewhere about a year after the accident, I found it described as "a devastating illness." It puzzled me. I had not considered my pain as an illness—but then I asked one of my pain specialists about my prognosis. The pain had become more chronic but had not yet reached the stage where I felt despair, as happened later on. I was still counting on a cure. I told him I planned to take early retirement and do development work abroad. What did he think? He shook his head. "You can't do that with your illnesses," he said. "You need to stay close to good doctors and good hospitals." Illnesses! I was not ill! I just had pain. Surely, someone, somehow, would cure me. And here he was telling me of my "illnesses." His words still echo in my mind. They signaled a turning point in my understanding of my problems and the beginning of the realization there might never be a cure. That the pain pointed to something very serious, something threatening my life as I knew it.

As time went on, the intensity, frequency, and duration of the pain kept increasing. I had to take sick leave, after which I tried to go back to work with the help of an assistant. I couldn't do it. The pain was slowly destroying me. Soon I had to take more sick leave, during which my doctors declared me unable to go back to work.

What was this intense pain like?

The following describes a *typical* morning during the worst four-year stretch, from 1999 to the end of 2003. I wake from a drug-induced sleep with my neck in spasm and a stabbing pain above my left eye. It is 4:30 a.m. Not aware yet of anything but the pain and the need to sleep, I move my head in the hope it will go away. It doesn't. I turn to my other side. It does not go away. What I must do is get out of bed, take medicine, and move my neck to slowly stretch the tissues that the night has turned to steel. But my body can't. My mind won't move. I am so deeply tired that I stay in bed, intensely aware of the pain. I fall asleep for a short while. I will never be able to explain this phenomenon I would not have considered possible, that is, that I sleep fully aware of the pain. A dual state that splits me in two, a splitting that itself demands such intense energy that I cannot maintain it for long.

I must massage the swelling in my neck. I stuff a small pillow under my upper left arm for support so I can reach the left side of my neck without having to hold my arm up. Just touching the swollen tissue sharply increases the pain. But I know I must. The only way out of the pain is to go right into it and through it. I am pushing out the debris that is stuck in inflamed tissues and presses on the nerves. I want to stop this torment and go back to sleep. I have to tell myself: keep going, keep at it. The pain does not go away. I shift my position, and momentarily the pain seems to pull back a bit. I sleep for a few seconds. Please God, let me sleep. The pain surges up again. My hand reaches for my neck once more. My fingers are tired. I use my right hand instead, reaching my arm across my chest to reach the left side. I can reach it, but it is too hard to do for long. I knew that—but it is always a last attempt at gaining a few more seconds of rest before I know that I have no choice but to get up. Then the hard work begins.

My head shakes itself clear of this need to sleep. I push myself up, shaking from pain and exhaustion. It is just before 5 a.m. I take medicine. I work myself into old warm house pants and a warm sweater. Nothing about me is presentable. Just as well I live alone. Going down the stairs blinded by pain, I hold on to the walls, fearing I might slip. I go for my La-Z-Boy, bought for this very purpose. Soft, yet sturdy, it provides extra lumbar support. The chair is wide. Enough room for my elbows. It rocks. I can get in and out easily. It swivels. I can turn the chair to look to the side and keep my head straight. Always keep my head straight.

It is still pitch dark outside. I manage to make coffee—quickly, putting a small filter on a cup. Coffee gives me the kick necessary to sit there in the dark and work on my neck. I light a candle on a small table next to the chair to comfort me with its flickering light. I will stay in that chair for a long time. I meditate. I center myself. I scream. I mumble: "God, please, let this pass. Please. I cannot do this anymore." He or She does not listen. I am so exhausted that my head falls forward. Not good. It stretches the tissues too suddenly and too far. I must hold up my head with inflamed muscles and with ligaments that no longer work.

I take more medicine. Tylenol 3, two of them, as well as Toradol (a non-steroidal anti-inflammatory drug or NSAID). And I'll take more in an hour or so if I need to. I have Percocet (oxycodone and acetaminophen) and M-Eslon (morphine) in the house but stay away from them as long as I can. Their side effects are intolerable. Between the drugs and cautiously moving my head, stretching it forward and to the side, massaging the neck again and again—the pain will settle to where, by late morning, I can start functioning. When I say the pain "settles" I do not mean it goes away. It means the steeliness has softened. That the worst is over for now. But the pain often stays all day. Floating in and out. I fear going to bed for fear of waking up.

During the worst four years, almost anything could trigger the pain: lifting objects, carrying things for even short distances, loud noises, loud voices, pop music (that beat!), television, city noise, being in a crowd, hurrying, turning my head to the side for more than two seconds, reaching sideways, driving, reading with my head bent down. Often I suffered a pain attack and had no idea what triggered it.

It could flare up anywhere. When I tried to continue teaching, the pain often flared up badly in the middle of class. Invariably, I had to end class early, lock myself in my office, and lie still on the floor for a long time till I could trust myself to drive home. In grocery stores, the pain would often flare up intensely (too many stimuli, bad music). I would abort the shopping, take medicine, sit in my car until the pain had settled enough to allow me to drive. Fear began to take over my days. During the worst years, I did not dare to go anywhere by myself further than half an hour away from home.

During the third year, a swelling starts in the middle of my neck just left of the spine. It feels like a large marble, round and hard. It can swell up for days, then shrink again. It always feels hard, and it hurts when pressed on. Right around it "electricity" gathers, and the lightest rubbing of the skin sets off fireworks. I try to bear it as long as possible, as the only way to get rid of that painful electricity is to work through it. Over the years I have received a dizzying array of contradictory diagnoses which, using my doctors' words, I list in chapter 4. I refer to this "thing" in my neck now as a "glob." That is as good a definition as any.

The first-year flare-ups often lasted a few days, after which I had a few days without any pain at all. Then the pain became worse and more chronic. The entire left side of my neck, left shoulder, and upper arm would turn into a tormenting trap. I think I now understand a little of the madness that animals experience when caught in steel traps. I often wished I could take a knife and *cut* right through the muscles where the neck ends and the shoulder begins, just as animals try to chew off their paws to get free. Many times, if only a doctor had said, "I can cut off your arm and that will be the solution," I would have said "Please! Do it! Now!" I fully understand Scott Fishman, who says of his patients in severe chronic pain that they will do anything to get rid of the pain, even risking total paralysis or death.[1]

I tried to describe this torment to my doctors and could not find the words to do so. Would they miss something important if I could not find the right words? What were the right words? I filled out the McGill Pain Questionnaire for various doctors. This is a list of seventy-eight pain descriptors: stabbing, burning, crawling, stinging, dull, sharp, piercing, frightful, terrifying, scalding, and a whole lot more. That helped. Yet, I always felt, in the short time we had, I was not adequately describing what was happening to me. In the worst years, when the pain stabbed me everywhere, I'd lie on the floor like a corpse. Hours would pass with nothing but stabbing piercing pain. Medication would barely have an effect. How could I speak about all that? My journal speaks for me:

June 2003. A horrid day, again, and again. Total depletion. Got up at 3 a.m. with pain on both sides of my neck and a stabbing head pain. About a dozen pills today. My mind is groggy. I never, never will be able to put the terror of this on paper. Couldn't bear to go outside and see nature's beauty. I stepped outside just for a moment and couldn't bear it. Tonight the depression hits suddenly. I sob from one moment to the next. The soup I was tasting spurts out of my mouth. Besides "managing" the pain, feeding the cats, and warming up some soup, I haven't been able to do anything today.

Then a friend gave me an article from the *New York Times* by Melanie Thernstrom, a journalist who spent time in a pain clinic in Boston.[2] Every paragraph had me in tears. Finally, words that spoke to what I was going through. This was me. I was not crazy. I was not exaggerating. Thernstrom described how constant pain did the kind of things to others that I was experiencing: the despair, the fear, the isolation, the terror. The doctors quoted in the article were my doctors: essentially helpless. In the words of a pain clinic director, "Some of my patients are on the border of human life. Chronic pain is like water damage to a house—if it goes on long enough, the house collapses." On the border of human life. That's where I lived during those worst years, one hour at the time.

Thernstrom notes how patients are often stumped by their doctor's request to describe their pain. They struggle for metaphors: "It's like being slammed into the wall and totally destroyed....There is nothing I can do to defend myself." That is the terrifying thing. Being without defenses. I lie completely still when the worst pain hits. No movement. Not of the body, not of the mind. The slightest movement anywhere spreads the pain everywhere. There is nothing I can do. As Thernstrom puts it, pain is "like the work of a torturer who must have—but won't reveal—a purpose." A good friend wrote, "This is how I imagine your pain...as a sadistic lover intent on forcing your compliance through whatever tortures can be devised, providing no expectation of relief or reward for you being responsive to every demand. It requires that you relinquish all power and choice in order to focus on how to accommodate the demands of pain, with no hope for ease or balance."

I sent Thernstrom's article along with a Christmas card to my two pain specialists, thanking them for their care. I told them that the article said much better than I could what the pain experience was like. On my next visit, one of them thanked me immediately—he really wanted to make me better and suffered from not being able to do so. The other specialist didn't remember. Oh, yes—he thought he had read it after all, but he did not remember the details. I know doctors are busy. But when I tell them, "This explains my pain better than I can myself," I think they need to read it. Pain is so difficult to talk about, yet a doctor can only rely on what the patient says. As Scott Fishman notes, pain is what the patient says it is.[3] But can the patient really say what it is?

One day, however (as I recorded in a June 2002 journal entry), I woke up with no pain—a very rare occurrence:

> I feel I am experiencing a miracle! I move my head carefully. I sit up slowly. Often sitting up or turning over sets off the pain. But not today! I lie down again carefully. Then, slowly, bit by bit, I sink into gratitude. Oh, my God, I am *so* grateful. Grateful to wake up to no pain! Relief sinks into my body. Tension leaves me. All the tissues of my body, mind, and emotions sink into a deep kind of rest. The relief is astonishing. My soul relaxes. It may be a normal morning! Pain is now what everything else is compared against. Pain is the master. When the pain mercifully stays away, I feel as if an abusive husband has left. As if a war has ended. As if a hurricane has finally passed.

"When the pain mercifully stays away…" The first time that phrase came into my head, I knew I no longer truly owned my own home. Thank you, Pain, for staying away. The pain has taken on the power of an active agent, a force that decides on its own when it enters my house and when it leaves. I don't scold it anymore. I bow toward it. I don't dare to curse it because to do so might enrage it to the point where it would return the next morning with an even greater force. It has become an expected, regular visitor, but the time of arrival and the length of its stay remain a secret. Therein lies much of its tyranny.

Who am I? Who was I? Who can I still be?

At first, I was the same person, whether in pain or not. I was convinced the pain would somehow disappear. Another few weeks, a few months perhaps. I would find the right doctor. I would come upon the right treatment. Pain or no pain, I was the same Lous. It was just a matter of waiting this out. But then I noticed something strange taking place. By the time the pain became hellish, a different person started to form itself inside the one I thought I was. Who is she? She scares me. Looking in the mirror when she turns up, I hardly recognize her as myself. She looks old, drawn, and pale. I don't understand her intrusion. What switches life from the Lous I know to this new person, or back again, is no more, but no less, than the onset or the stopping of intense pain. It is like an electrical switch. From the light to the dark. Or the other way around. Nothing is the same in these two different worlds. To this day, I still cannot explain these alternate worlds in which I now live, and in each one of which I am a different person. I think I now have a sense of what it may be like to live as a split personality: I have developed one, for reasons different than those understood in the world of psychiatry, but I am split nevertheless.

As the months passed and the pain got worse, this other person who began as an intruder gradually became the familiar one. The one most often present. The one who obliterates the past, torments the present, and makes the future unbearable before the fact. Bit by bit, it has become almost impossible for me to remember who I once was. A health-care professional interviewed by Arthur Rosenfeld put it this way: "Chronic pain is an unimaginable destructive experience, destructive to our sense of self. It demoralizes people. It breaks their spirit....It can lead to suicide. I have patients who have suffered ten or fifteen years of chronic pain, and they are shadows of their former selves."[4]

I would look at pictures of myself taken in the years before the accident and have a hard time remembering "her" as myself. The pictures showed a young and energetic-looking woman. I had done all these things I was doing in the photo. Been to all those places. But by the time the pain was at its worst, I had become someone else. "A crumbled woman," is how one of my daughters described me. A strange shadow of my former self. Yet, I have an intimate knowledge of this person in the picture. I know how she thought, felt, loved, walked, and worked. The kind of mother she was. I know the shades of her emotions. I understand how her mind worked. I like this woman. I want to be her. How did she slip through my fingers?

During those worst years, and often still, tears well at the slightest incident: beautiful music, a sentimental film, a sensitive word from someone, a insensitive word from someone, and I fall apart just when I think I have myself under control. A kind word, or just the right question from a doctor or from my therapist, and there I go. The tensions in this life in pain are always just right under the surface. Who am I? Who can I still be? How can I still be somebody?

Chaos and the Difficulty of Telling

Arthur Frank stresses the healing that results from writing one's story of illness and suffering.[5] In *The Wounded Storyteller,* he shows how the person who turns illness into story transforms fate into experience. As wounded persons, he says, they may be cared for, but as storytellers, they care for others by creating empathetic bonds between themselves and their listeners, and by recovering the voices that illnesses and pain often take away. But, he warns, telling does not come easy, and neither does listening.

It does not come easy for those living with chronic pain, because pain eats away one's energy and erases one's thoughts. In August 2002 I wrote, "I am so tired, so wiped out and in turmoil, in so much pain, my head so heavy, my feelings both numb and explosive, that all I can think of is folding up in bed and staying there forever."

Another reason Frank cites for the difficulty of telling is the nature of language itself that prevents the chaos of severe illness and pain to be told. There must be distance from the chaos to allow for the reflection necessary to do the writing. Writing itself forces order onto chaos, but it cannot capture it. Making the attempt to capture chaos in language means leaving chaos behind. Scribbling hundreds of pages of notes offered me a mode of survival, in part, I am sure, because of the ordering process demanded by language. Such ordering on my part provided the anchor that kept me from falling off the edge of life.

Chaos has an order all its own: an order that appears at the conscious level only as utter and sustained bewilderment. Does chaos find a home somewhere? Can it be told in some form away from language? Art may be one way. Edvard Munch's famous painting *The Scream* of the woman on a bridge does it for me. But art is not a vehicle everyone finds accessible. There is, however, one form of experience available to everyone that leaves the chaos of the waking hours intact while telling about it in an alternate form. It is dreams and nightmares.

In *The Wounded Storyteller,* Frank does not mention the dreamworld. He writes a conscious human narrative, while dreams are narratives issued directly from the unconscious, without mediation by the ordering properties of thought and language. Without any concern for the order of time, place, reason, or any of the other spatial and temporal dimensions of our waking hours. The numerous nightmares I had in those years of severe and constant pain told a striking narrative of the chaos my life had become.

Seeing chronic pain as a nightmare is not a metaphorical exercise. It offers a descriptor, the essence of which David Morris captures well:

> Nightmare is not simply a figure of speech when applied to chronic pain. Lawrence LeShan, from the Institute of Applied Biology, described the universe perceived by the patient in chronic pain as structurally identical with the universe of the nightmare. Nightmares, according to LeShan, possess three unvarying features: (1) terrible things are being done and worse are threatened; (2) we are helplessly under the control of outside forces; and (3) we cannot predict when the ordeal will end. Leshan concludes: "The person in pain is in the same formal situation: terrible things are being done to him and he does not know if worse will happen; he has no control and is helpless to take effective action; no time limit is given." Only one feature should be added to LeShan's description. Chronic pain is a nightmare from which we may never truly awaken—or a waking state in which the nightmare never ends.[6]

Given the ordering of experience demanded by language there is no point in talking about these dreams. I must relate the images the way I wrote them down, almost feverishly, on awakening. Here are a few of them, chosen almost at random:

> I am traveling. Ton [my sister] will take me to the airport. One suitcase is already in her car. I am trying to pack a second suitcase. I need to hurry. But the clothes in my closet are not mine; they belong to Miep [my other sister]. I ask her where in the hell my things are. She says she wanted my closet for her own clothes. I yell at her. She should never have changed things without asking me. My cousin appears. He tells me to hurry, otherwise I'll miss the plane. I get even more nervous. I can't find what I am looking for. I feel I'm going crazy. Somehow I pack another suitcase and run outside and into my cousin's car. Ton's car has already left, and I can see it just at the end of the street. I want to follow her, but my cousin says, no, we are going a quicker way. I panic. We will lose Ton. We will never meet each other, and I will miss the plane. I wake up.

> I am across from the house where I was raised, sitting on a large stone, without clothes. I am cold, hungry, and tired. I so badly want to go inside, but no one lets me in. The window is open, and I see my sister who is doing

something to my mother's blouse. Neither is aware that I am locked outside, cold and hungry. I feel abandoned. I have no home. Then Aunt Anne comes out of the house and puts her arm around my shoulders, saying, "I am so sorry, it must be terrible to be in such pain." Then she is gone, and I am still outside, staring with tears in my eyes at the window where I can still see my mother and sister. I wake up.

I am in a large city. I have to teach. I can't find the building. I walk down a narrow street and suddenly see the university. There are several doors and I don't know which one is the right one. I enter one at random and find myself in a huge hall with corridors leading off in all directions. I fall and drop my books. I pick them up and hurry blindly down one of the corridors. I don't recognize any of the classrooms. I turn around and head in the opposite direction. Suddenly I see some students whom I recognize and a door with my name on it. I am almost there. I fall. My books are scattered all over the floor. I wake up.

I am in a doctor's office. He seems like a nice man. But after a few minutes his face turns hollow and corpselike. He asks me to sit next to him and suddenly puts his head in my lap. I am stunned. He says, "Oh, come on." I freeze. Suddenly there is another man, older and creepy looking. He takes my arm and stretches it out for the ugly doctor. I think he is going to cut into my arm. I can't get away. The door opens. It's the doctor who had his head in my lap, now looking fine, young, professional, carrying a file. He is with another nice-looking man. I see my chance and run out the door. I wake up.

I am in a large city in China. I am lost. Someone stole my purse. I want to tell someone, but I can't speak Chinese. I am exhausted. I see a building with men in uniform at the door. One of them speaks English. I feel such relief. I tell him what happened. He smiles and says not to worry. He gives me a temporary Chinese passport and some Chinese money. He tells me that they will put me on a train back to England. It will be a rough ride. I may have to stand most of the way, but it will get me back. I am so relieved and grateful that I do not care. But I do think, "That will be hard on my neck. I will go into pain." I wake up.

Alone, in fear, vulnerable, cold, lost, losing things, unable to find my way, powerless, unable to do my work, in tears, in pain, exhausted, with a mother and sister who can't help, with doctors who don't know how to help and some that are outright abusive. The parallels to my waking life during the worst years are terrifying. My waking life *felt* just like these dreams.

Why me? Why not me?

September 2001. I am in the Toronto subway. The scene is not attractive. It is the afternoon rush hour and people look tired. Many seem to be staring at nothing, thinking God knows what. But they are not in pain. No one smiles. Few talk. But they are not in pain.

That morning brought a nice surprise: I only had a slight headache, which a Tylenol took care of. I ventured into town, treating myself to an early dinner. Something I had not been able to do for over a month. At the end of the dinner, however, my neck started to stiffen and become painful, and I needed to return home before it got worse. As I look at my fellow passengers on the subway, the thought comes to me as it so often has: I wish I were one of them. Any one of them. Nothing can be as bad as this constant pain. Self-pity intensifies. I begin to panic, thinking of all the tomorrows to come, and the pain spreads to my shoulders and back. The spot above my left eye is throbbing. I feel my eyes tearing. Why can't I be one of them? Why is this happening to me?

Often I tell myself that I'd trade my pain for deafness, for life in a wheelchair, for whatever. Anything but this constant pain. I have tried hard to imagine myself in such conditions. However difficult they might be, I could learn to live with them. I know I cannot learn to "live with" this pain—not for another twenty or thirty years. When I realize that this pain may never go away, my chest tightens and I can scarcely breathe.

Physicians Angela Mailis-Gagnon and David Israelson tell of a patient whose leg had become numb from his foot to just above the knee.[7] For eighteen years he walked with the help of a brace that helped him lift his foot off the ground. Then he fell and ended up with knee pain that, despite medications, got worse and worse while the numbness and paralysis went away completely. He pleads with his doctors to take away his pain and give him back the numbness and paralysis.

With chronic pain there is no prognosis. No doctor has ever mentioned when I might get better. Or if I ever will. During the worst four years I often wished the accident had ended my life. *Anything,* but these thousands of hours of pain. And the many more to come. James Henry cites research that shows that health-related quality of life of chronic pain noncancer patients is among the lowest observed for any medical condition.[8]

The comparisons I draw to other illnesses are not really meant to be true comparisons: they reflect an attempt to portray the severity of this insidious and invisible disease that many people do not even believe is real. Of course, I know that what some people live with is a greater hell than mine: torture, deep poverty, horrible terminal illnesses, ongoing rape. But during the worst years when pain was destroying me, my life was worse than anyone else's. I was sure of it.

Over time, however, I have started to ask myself the question: Why should I be exempt? When I think of all the others who suffer greatly, my agitated mind slows down. I sink into a field of belonging into which my soul is very slowly learning to settle.

Death

"Chronic pain is a long, long, slow death," a woman suffering from severe chronic pain told me. Elaine Scarry refers to "the kinship between pain and death, both of which are radical and absolute, found only at the boundaries they themselves create."[9] That pain is so often used as a symbolic substitute for the death of childhood in the initiation rites of many tribes is a recognition, says Scarry, that pain is the equivalent in felt experience of what is unfeelable in death: in each instance, the contents of consciousness dies. Severe physical pain always mimes death.

During my worst four years, every day resembled dying. Even now, I often feel strangely close to death. Not because of "ideations" of suicide, as my good doctor wrote in his report to another doctor, but because this life in pain has asked of me to part from nearly all that I thought constituted my life. Death as *afscheid nemen*. I have to say this in Dutch, my mother tongue, to capture what I mean. To say goodbye, to take leave in the deep sense of parting—parting for a long time, perhaps for ever, from people, from places, from activities that are very dear. This parting as an ongoing process often renders an aloneness that feels total and is so numbing that it brings on more despair and more pain. Isolation, and the taboo that slowly develops about talking about one's pain to others, intensifies inner turmoil and intensifies the pain itself. Dr. David Kuhl in *What Dying People Want* states that no one with serious uncontrollable pain ought to be left to experience it alone.[10] He was writing about the dying. Yet, experiencing intense pain alone often happens, hour after hour, week after week, year after year to those who suffer from severe chronic pain and who live alone.

In my many readings on chronic pain, only Marni Jackson mentions living alone as a major additional factor in suffering.[11] Living alone while in constant severe pain is a special form of hell. Assuming, of course, that a companion would be understanding and helpful—otherwise togetherness may well be a greater hell. As Jackson puts it, "Being loved can help us distinguish between mere pain and bottomless, free-fall suffering. This is why people in chronic pain who live alone are not just at the mercy of a body that hurts. Over time, their pain becomes inseparable from a larger sense of being unconsoled and (much worse) being inconsolable. Their pain becomes a voicing of their isolation."

My friend and I were going to go out for dinner and a movie. This friend, who I like very much, lived many miles away, and I had not seen her for several years. She was in town only for a short while. I was having a few decent days and looked forward to spending time with her. Then, the devil returned. The morning of our outing I was in terrible pain. No choice but to cancel. I called and told her my throbbing, stabbing head would not be able to tolerate a movie. I wanted her to come anyway, sit with me, and hold my hand, figuratively speaking. But I did not dare to ask. I heard myself being hesitant and vague, saying I could not go to the movie but perhaps a dinner at my house would be OK. Perhaps she could pick up some food on her way.

"Let's cancel," she said, "and you can stay home quietly." I am certain she thought she was doing me a favor. Had I been in her shoes I would have done the same: someone in great pain wouldn't be up for any visits and would prefer to be home alone, wouldn't she?

My heart sank. "I have been home quietly in pain now for years," I wanted to say. "I can't take it anymore. Please, come over and just sit with me." But they were the words I couldn't speak.

During the worst years of constant severe pain the feeling of abandonment was at first focused on being abandoned by particular people, and then it shifted to feeling abandoned by the universe itself. It felt total. Then, bit by bit, the feeling of abandonment shifted to something quite the opposite: the sense that the universe was begging me to come. I often felt I was walking its edge toward death. I longed for death's promise of rest and relief. Not to struggle out of bed anymore when pain wakes me in the midst of darkness for the umpteenth time, my neck swollen, my head stabbing. Not to have to dull myself with drugs. Death will be a liberator, leading me to a light, restful place, taking me elsewhere peacefully. Death appears kind to me, not like Pain, whom I imagine as a devil with raked horns. There is a certain beauty to death I never could have seen before. This pull toward death is not the same as thoughts of suicide. For those living with constant pain, suicide is the ultimate painkiller. When I think of suicide, it is not because I long for death but because I need this pain to end.

But here I am, preparing my protein shakes and juicing fresh vegetables to enhance my general health and stamina as much as possible—while my head is afloat in the desire to lie down and rest forever. My constant efforts to stay as healthy as possible, on the one hand, and my intense desire for eternal rest, on the other. Part of this split existence.

The Calendar

March 2002, still in Toronto. One of the worst years. The days on my calendar are now mostly blank, to be crossed off, one after the other. It seems I cross off far more days than I used to. There are the same number of days in a year, but I swear I cross off more of them. Because, when I do, it seems I just did. Nothing seems to have happened in between. Only pain. One week looks like another. One month looks like another. In the spaces for the weekdays are my medical appointments. I forget what month it is. April, October, February—it doesn't matter. I just received my death sentence from the pain specialist: "There is no cure. We are running out of options. Take morphine." My calendar, once filled with work engagements, family events, and dates with friends, may stay forever empty.

> As the body breaks down, it becomes increasingly the object of attention, usurping the place of all other objects, so that finally, in very very old and sick people, the world may exist only in a circle two feet out from themselves; the exclusive content of perception and speech may become what was eaten, the problems of excreting, the progress of pains, the comfort or discomfort of a particular chair or bed.[12]

Why do Scarry's words bring me to tears? I am not dying. I am not very old. Yet they describe the shrinkage of my life. My wonderful La-Z-Boy chair, bought especially to meet the pain each morning, is a major topic of conversation with my daughters, as are the many pillows I have tried out for my neck. On their visits they cook and freeze food so I don't have to attend to food preparation for several days. I perceive myself as very old and sick when pain reigns for days, for weeks. As I cross off a day, I feel I cross off something abstract. I don't know what I am crossing off because I wasn't there.

At times, I do put a fun thing on my calendar. A movie I want to see. A concert I want to go to. I read about them in the paper. I move into that space where I want to live again. I go alone, so I don't risk having to cancel on someone at the last moment. I can leave in the middle of the movie if I need to. I don't have to go out for a coffee afterward. Often, I cannot go. Pain or intense fatigue intervenes. It is quite an occasion when I do get to go. I dress nicely, the way I used to. Seeing myself in pajamas and old house clothes almost all the time, I hardly recognize myself. I look in the mirror and see someone I used to know. Someone I do remember, but she isn't me. I leave the house, almost nervous about feeling normal. Often it takes me close to an hour to get to where I need to go. I have had to return more than once when pain flares up before I get there. I have a concert penciled in for next month. I paid for the ticket. Will I be able to go? The calendar, once a daily friend that logged my busy days, now records my wiped out life.

Am I still normal?

It is May 2003 in Victoria, seven years after the accident. Life moves so slowly. One little thing at a time. Routine tasks I used to do quickly—doing dishes, shopping, cleaning, dressing, handling finances—now fill all my good hours. "Mum," one of my daughter says pensively and with a sad voice, "you're a different person. You used to do so much." A few weeks earlier I had written:

> The pain takes all of me. I look at the corner of the living room where there are about ten plants. Cat hair and dead leaves are between the plants. It badly needs vacuuming. That means moving the plants, cleaning up, and putting them all back. I will have to bend over, trying to keep my neck and

head straight. A big deal. Normally this would have taken me all of five minutes. But now pain is slobbering up my energy so fast and furiously that small tasks that once were nothing are now insurmountable.

I venture a dinner at my new home. My first social event since I arrived in Victoria. I invite two people who I got to know while looking for a house and establishing my medical life here. One of my daughters who lives in Olympia and who enjoys these things comes to help out. The morning is filled with pain, however, and she urges me to cancel. I don't want to. I long for a normal evening, to be social and forget about this constricted life of mine. With the help of Tylenols and Percocets I keep the pain under control. Half way through a very pleasant dinner, the pain flares up. Badly and piercing. For some ten minutes my mind manages to suppress the pain, making an agreeable response to what is being said. Not my style. I massage my neck and shoulder. Who am I kidding to think they don't notice? But no one says a thing. The dinner goes right on, as if nothing happened. Yet everyone there knew I was in pain. Denying the presence of pain that evening reflected what chronic pain sufferers routinely experience: after a while people act as if nothing is the matter. You yourself act as if nothing is the matter. What is there to say? For my part, my inner voice was telling me that my pain must not interfere with other people's pleasures.

That evening I excused myself, hoping that if I could just lie down, take another Percocet, and stretch my neck, I could get the pain back under control. I left the table and lay down on my bed. My eyes got teary. I so much wanted a "normal" evening. The pain became intense as I lay there, lonelier than ever, hearing the voices of my guests at the table. Then I suddenly felt far away. In the company of others who were in pain, wherever they might be.

I decided later I should have acted differently. I should have stayed. I could have simply told my guests the pain was bad and I needed to stretch out on the couch. One of them could have massaged my neck. Their concern could have relaxed me. I would have felt part of the group. But, instead, we all took part in excluding me.

It is now August 2003. The sun shines gloriously. I'm having a decent day and decide to take a walk to the pond on the property. The ground is very uneven and is covered with high grass. I like the look of wildness. But I can't see where I am placing my feet. Around me are large moss-covered rocks, so characteristic of Vancouver Island. I walk dangerously in this happy moment, the water in the pond reflecting the sun's rays. I feel free in my movements the way I walked before the accident. Somewhere in my mind is a warning: I hear the voice of my first specialist, who told me that I would be in great pain for the rest of my life and then added, "And do not fall. Do not have another accident. Don't walk on uneven ground."

I venture a jump. A small one. From one rock to another. I ignore my ankles that feel a bit wobbly. So out of practice. All goes well. I feel so normal. A few days later I do it again. I am a bit more daring and jump from a rock onto the ground. I feel as if I am flying again! I feel free! This time the landing goes wrong. I feel the vertebrae in my neck shift. Inexorably, sharp pain flares up and lasts for days. Yet, I have no regrets. The yearning to do something normal, something that used to bring such joy, to recapture, even if only for a minute, that feeling of lightness and adventure without considering the consequences—I had to do it.

I had a doctor's appointment a few days later and was still in serious pain. He asked if I knew what triggered it. I shrugged, so I wouldn't have to explicitly lie about it. I knew he would not have approved of my jumping stones. How can I explain to a doctor that, just once in a while, no matter the consequences, I need to act normal to stay sane?

Rooting the Self in the Present

I force myself to stay here, now. With this moment. It is December 10, 2003. I just woke up to stabbing pain. I make coffee. Holding my head up with my hands, pushing against the swollen tissue. I feed the cats. Time for Tylenol 3 and Toradol. I just sit, massaging my neck muscles that the night has turned to steel. I absorb my purring three-legged stray cat, now so tame, curled up on the couch. The beauty of the surroundings. The fields. The trees. This quiet place. I feel a sense of happiness, even as I sit there with a stabbing headache, fingers pushing against my swollen neck muscles.

"How can you be happy?" my inner voice asks. I am having thoughts again. I am no longer attending to the moment. I don't even know if I will be able to manage to take the ferry to Olympia to be with my daughter for Christmas. Pain like this would make it impossible to go. How can it be

I feel something resembling happiness? Every morning I wake up to devil-ish pain, and I never know how long it will last or how often it will flare back up during the day. How can I plan anything that way? How can I live that way?

I do live that way. It has started to rain. Two young deer are on my drive-way. They cross the driveway to the grass and graze, as always so gracefully—an impressionist painting taking shape before my eyes. The rain falling around the deer makes the world glimmer and tremble. The here and now is back. The Brahms violin concerto on the radio comes to that place some-where in the middle where it soars. My cat softly blinks his eyes at me. Hap-piness is back, right here, as long as I stay in the present, in this moment.

There are only moments. Tomorrow, next year are ideas. Projections. Not reality. When I think of the future, my life is indeed ruined. But here is Brahms, the deer, my cat's soft eyes. The pain, dulled by Tylenol 3s and Toradol, is now under some control. The moment is what it is. It sounds so intellectually appealing. For me it is a matter of survival. For thoughts about both the past and future are terrible threats. But easy it is not.

"Have you ever noticed that your awareness of pain is not in pain even when you are?" asks Jon Kabat-Zinn, founding director of the Stress Re-duction Clinic at the University of Massachusetts Medical Center, in *Com-ing to Our Senses,* his book on mindfulness meditation.[13] It's a critically important observation, and one that is relatively easy to make when pain is light. Now and then, even when in severe pain, I can move into that present state just for a second or two, and my awareness of the pain, indeed, is not in pain. It is a strange, liberating feeling. I am up here somewhere, and this torturous pain is down there somewhere. It is like falling into peace.

When tormenting pain is constant, however, awareness of the pain, as distinct from the pain itself, is extremely difficult to maintain. It slips away. It is nearly impossible to imagine how severe physical pain grabs one's attention and blots out thought, erasing one's ability to give direction to awareness. It would take the power of attentiveness of the Buddha himself to be grounded continually in moment-to-moment awareness of the pres-ent. Under the weight of severe ongoing pain, the scope of one's attentive-ness is profoundly altered: tomorrows and yesterdays blur into one long stretched out here and now of pain. The separation between different time zones starts to collapse. The boundaries thought draws between hours and hours, days and days, and between days and nights start to slowly dissolve. Severe constant pain pulls attentiveness forcefully into the moment, not into awareness of the moment (that, one has to do deliberately), but into the ongoing moment of the direct, concrete pain experience.

Speaking of the awareness of pain not being in pain even though you are, Kabat-Zinn puts it this way:

> If you move into pure awareness in the midst of pain, even for the tiniest moment, your relationship with your pain is going to shift right in that very moment. It is impossible for it not to change because the gesture of holding it, even if not sustained for long, even for a second or two, already reveals its larger dimensionality.[14]

It can be done, but indeed, for most of us, not for long, he seems to say. Though he may also be implying that these moments, though only moments, have a transforming and lasting effect. That, I find to be true—now that the pain has lessened in intensity and frequency.

It is now April 2006, and the prolotherapy and wellness approaches to the pain have brought about a distinct improvement. I do not dare to think whether these occasional moments of "awareness of my pain that itself is not in pain" would have had a lasting effect had the pain continued in its hellish form—I fear I would have drowned.

It is not as straightforward as it sounds then, this staying in the present when suffering from constant pain, for Pain itself takes charge of thought and time—collapsing them into one long moment that seamlessly reproduces itself. The long moment takes on the sameness of the blank pages in my calendar. Says Arthur Frank, "When we are in great pain…eternity has a way of opening up under us, and over us and to the side of us."[15] Emily Dickinson, too, understood this:

> Pain—has an Element of Blank—
> It cannot recollect
> When it begun—if there were
> A time when it was not—
> It has no Future—but itself—
> Its Infinite realms contain

> Its Past—enlightened to perceive
> New Periods—of Pain.[16]

In the domain of chronic pain there is no future different from chronic pain. There is no doctor who, with certainty, can promise otherwise.

Can this suffering be mitigated? In the end I must agree with Kabat-Zinn: if there is anything at all, it is staying rooted in the here and now. There is no other way. No matter how difficult it is to do and how often you fail. You must go back to awareness of the moment, again and again. This requires a deliberate, disciplined approach, for mindfulness is not just an attitude. At the end of the residential program at the Victoria Pain Clinic, I ask Michael Greenwood, the clinic's medical director and himself a daily meditator, "How does one live this way?" His answer is immediate: "A life of meditation." That is all he says. "A life of being in the present," he could have said. I know he is right. When in constant pain, it is just such a long, long present.

Eric Cassell, in *The Nature of Suffering*, says that suffering ends if the person can be promised that the pain will come to an end.[17] Acute pain hurts, but it does not cause suffering because you know it will go away. You just have pain for a short while. I clearly remember saying in great despair to my therapist in Toronto, "Give me more pain, worse pain even...for a month, a year—as long as I know it will be over after that. Then I can bear it." She nodded but didn't say a word. When no one can promise an end to suffering, says Cassell, doctors should try to be "causing" the sufferers to root themselves in the absolute present. Unfortunately, he notes, that is difficult to accomplish. Indeed. Only the person herself or himself can do that. But doctors certainly can encourage it once they themselves understand what it involves.

In my case, the realization of what "being in the present" meant came one day with sharp clarity: the only way to escape past and future terrors is not to go there. Just do not go there. Stay here. No matter what the here involves. With a recognition coming from a place I did not know existed, I saw that "here" is the only place where I really *can* be. "This is it." Only this. Now. This pain above my left eye. This thought. This fear. The beauty of this music. The softness of this fur purring against me. This steel in my neck. This lying awake.

Gradually, I have been able to go into the "this" state a bit more easily. Still, major pain attacks throw me back into terror, telling me that each day of the years that are left of my life the monster can return, take me into its mouth and crunch me. I still lose it when my thoughts go there, and I reach for the Valium. But I have started to breathe easier when in pain by staying with the "this." Just sitting. Just looking at the trees outside. Just going to some center in my body. Just listening to music. This, this, and this. Slowly, some healing started to slip into this present. In the words of cancer surgeon Balfour Mount, "Healing occurs in the present moment."[18] Healing occurs not in relation to a past we remember, or a future we project. Healing is a dynamic in the present.

I learned that staying rooted in the present involves still another difficulty: letting go of the intense desire—though not necessarily the possibility thereof—to be cured. It may well be the most difficult demand in being present and therefore also of healing. It's the entanglement and obsession involved in the desire for a future cure that stands in the way. One's intention needs to be to be in the present. Period. If the intention is to get rid of pain, one cannot empty the desiring and worrying mind and be in the here and now. I figure, if trying to get rid of the pain worked, by now my twenty some doctors and specialists would have figured out how to go about it.

Rooting the self in the here and now has made it possible for me to maintain some sense of coherence and sanity in the face of constant pain. Beyond that, it has brought moments of peace and beauty in ways I could not have imagined possible.

Beauty

It is January 2004. I take a shortcut through Bolen Books to get to my optometrist's office, and my eye catches the title of a book on display—*Beauty: The Invisible Embrace,* by John O'Donohue.[19] Drawn to the title, I open the book at random: "Beauty does not linger, it only visits. Yet beauty's visitation affects us and invites us into its rhythm." Then Donohue writes something that pierces my pained heart, and I buy the book immediately based on these few words:

A life without delight is only half a life. Lest this be construed as a plea for decadence or a self-indulgence that is blind to the horrors of the world, we should remember that beauty does not restrict its visitations only to those whom fortune or circumstance favour. Indeed, it is often the whispers and glimpses of beauty which enable people to endure on desperate frontiers. Even, and perhaps especially, in the bleakest times, we can still discover and awaken beauty; these are precisely the times when we need it most.

The young deer, the first one that came close to the house after I moved here, all grace and curiosity, now visits daily. The morning finds him waiting for his free breakfast of birdseed or apples. When the snow storm—all of about one inch of soft snow—visited us for two days, he slept on the porch against the front door of the house, sheltered from the harsh wind. When I first saw him less than half a year ago, his young body was fuzzy and of a deep bronze color. His long legs, a dancing grace. His eyes, velvety brown, looking curiously at me from a safe distance. I called him "Beauty." He brings a healing power whenever he walks into my backyard. Always on his time. Expected, yet unexpected. He comes. He goes. As true beauty, he just visits. Beauty stands there, now no more than a few meters away. He gazes at me. He takes me in. The pain softens as I absorb his velvet eyes, the soft lines of his flank, the playful circling of his tail. At ease, Beauty steps away. In the middle of the yard he stops, bends his hind legs and lets go of his bowels. That too, he does with unaffected grace. He walks on, taking some of my difficult life with him.

Something is stirred in me by Beauty's hovering presence. He spreads out the pain, thins it, lightens it, and transforms some of it into a softness that ripples away into the nature that surrounds us. Into something beyond myself that nevertheless holds me.

Beauty. It is a miracle to me that in all this pain beauty still comes. And it is more important to me now than ever. "In the cut and thrust of life experience," says Donohue, "beauty frequently emerges when either great love or great sacrifice elevates an experience above its daily confines to another level of presence and possibilities."[20] Beauty has lost all of its romanticism for me or its connection to sensuality. It now goes deeper and wider. To spaces hollowed by pain and loneliness, vessels for beauty, filled in fuller measure than it ever could before.

Music

Daniel Barenboim is playing Chopin's nocturnes. The pain has been so bad all morning. The moment I hear the first notes of the nocturne in E flat major, I am engulfed by something larger than me. Instantly. "You are safe now," it whispers, "you can let yourself go....I will hold you." My hyped-up nervous system quiets down. My attention goes to something I could never produce myself, yet is so deeply of myself. The music fills me up the way extreme pain does. But it brings a stillness rather than agony. It fills me to that point where nothing else exists. Where someone's voice would be an intrusion. Someone's touch a distraction. The music comes as grace. Severe pain and utter beauty, how can they merge? For that short while, they do. The pain is there, but it is not there. Then, Chopin passes.

I have been in awe of the effect of music from the first time the pain was altered by it. The commonality between intense pain and utter beauty, I suddenly thought, is that both command the present. Both intense pain and beauty exist on their own terms. In the here and now only. Nor is there a consciously fashioned language to pin them down.

I highlight the nocturne on the jacket. I know it is what I want to have played at my funeral. "Nocturne" means "night piece." I am moved by the appropriateness of the word "night" as my thoughts go to my funeral. I carefully pick out two others I love: the one in B major and the one in E minor. I highlight those on the jacket as well, while I look at Chopin's vulnerable, intense face on the CD cover. What did he know and feel? Can listening to his music bring about the same knowing, the same feelings out of which it came? Perhaps it can.

What is it in Chopin's music that makes me think of my death? I see clarity in it, an expression of thoughts and emotions simultaneously, before they ever got separated. A unity of life and death. For me, only Mozart rises to or above that nocturne's lucidity. Mozart, too, I want at my funeral. Perhaps the beauty of music connects me to my death because it makes me yearn for the fullness of life that has slipped so far away from me that often I have no memory of it.

Music reaches me with an immediacy that takes me by surprise. Before I know it, the music has already taken me in. It reaches into the pain and then transcends it. It does not "kill" or "dull" pain, as medications do. It works in a different way. It engulfs pain and takes it up into another sphere. John O'Donohue says it well: "The mystery of music is its uncanny ability to coax harmony out of contradiction and chaos....It is as though the music instinctively knows where you dwell and what you need....Music is often the only language which can find those banished to the nameless interior of illness."[21] Music indeed finds me there.

Nature

It is seven years since the accident. A chiropractic adjustment has resulted in a flaming pain attack. Tylenol 3 does nothing. I do not want to go to the Percocet. I do not like my mind played with, which it tends to do. I try the obnoxiously expensive triptan Imitrex first. Made for migraines, it helps sometimes better than Tylenol 3. But I can't have more than two in twenty-four hours. Later on in the day I need Percocet after all. Sleep only comes with sleeping pills. This goes on for five days. Another drugged out, desperately dark week.

This sunny morning the worst finally broke. I am intensely aware of the fear I felt the last few days: This is it. It will never get better. I failed at staying rooted in the present. I panicked. Still in pain, I go and sit outside. I am depleted. It is mid-November, but in front of the house out of the wind, the sun brings new warmth after weeks of rain and storm. I rest. Rest. The sun spills over my face. Unbelievably, I feel joy.

The large buck suddenly appears from between the small trees and bushes on the other side of the driveway. The size of a small horse, this huge beautifully antlered creature stands motionless, looking at me. A young fawn appears and darts gracefully around him. The little one is a frequent visitor who comes close to the house, intrigued by my cats, unafraid. The buck is now closer than ever before. My young cat starts creeping up on the little one.

The sun. This buck standing there, looking so attentively at me. The young deer darting around it. My young cat sneaking up to it. The wild and the domesticated, fascinated by each other. Their curiosity gets the best of the young deer and the cat. They seek each other out. The young deer lifts its head toward her. Its eyes focus, its ears prick up, its spindly legs dance toward the cat. The cat pretends to charge him. Just a few steps. Then she stretches out and walks calmly away. The young deer walks after her, coming up to her to almost touching distance. They walk down the driveway together and disappear into the bushes. I watch spellbound as the edges of pain blur and soften. For a short time, all threatening thoughts of the future are gone.

This is not the kind of distraction that books on pain often advise, such as watching TV, a trip to the mall, chatting with a friend—all legitimate means to distraction from pain, from mild pain that is. For when severe pain strikes they don't work for me. Then distractions increase pain. They do not transcend the pain into something else. Kabat-Zinn, in *Full Catastrophe Living*, says much the same thing.[22] Instead of using distractions to escape from pain, he asks us to bring mindfulness meditation *to* the pain and to stay rooted in the present.

Here in the sun, the buck, the wild playing with the tame, the wonder of their disappearance, side by side, into the bushes—it works in a totally different way than do distractions. I cannot summon this beauty, as I can distractions. It appears unasked, always as a grace, as a blessing. Beauty lifts me into itself for a timeless moment, into a still point, where there are *no* distractions. Where there is only pure attentiveness. Pain has gone to the buck, to the little one, to the trees. It slipped away from me as all my attention went to that wild other, bringing a moment of total rest. Of surrendering these things called "I" and "pain." Bringing a meaning I only hesitantly refer to as "happiness." I think of it as happiness of a certain kind. A special kind I cannot yet put into words. It is at the core of attention. It is as ephemeral as it is real. It holds no space for fear. No doctor can treat me in that manner. It cannot be bought at the drugstore. I want to hold on to it, but can't. Holding on to beauty is a contradiction in terms. The buck and the fawn have walked out of my view. But they are around. After distractions, I often feel emptier, and the quality of the pain returns just the same. But this magical scene wove me into something larger than myself. The pain is there, but it has been blessed, in a manner of speaking. For days afterward, the pain does not weigh so heavily on me.

4 *Pain and the World of Pain Management*

Introducing My Medical Life

My doctors and other health-care workers. In how many ways do I know them? There have been the gentle ones. The rude ones. The attentive ones. The nonlistening ones. The truly caring ones. The clearly uncaring ones. The humble ones. The arrogant ones. The broadly informed ones. The narrowly trained ones. The ones who have no time for you. The ones who try to have time for you.

I think I have started to pick up early signs of what lies ahead when meeting a new doctor. Their eyes—whether they look straight at you with interest, or whether they stay focused on what is in your file. Their body language—whether it is welcoming, or rushed and rigid. Their choice of words—are they all fact oriented, or is there a sense of kindness? Do they shake your hand when they first greet you? Do you feel at ease when you speak, or do you wonder whether they are actually listening to what you are trying to say? When you have left their office, do you barely remember what was said, or do you feel that someone is now on your side and is going to help you, one way or the other?

I have seen twenty-two doctors and specialists, as well as many alternative health-care workers as a direct consequence of the accident. In all, I have encountered over sixty health-care professionals in eleven years. This large number is mainly the result of endless referrals, the need for second opinions, the many different pain problems and syndromes that developed over time necessitating still another kind of professional, and the fact that finding a doctor, specialist, or alternative professional who can help in your specific case is largely a matter of trial and error.

Scott Fishman has noted that by the time patients arrive at his clinic, they have sought help from multiple doctors at numerous hospitals and clinics.[1] And despite batteries of tests and an exhausting stream of medications, he says, the suffering continues while they clash with a new adversary: a medical culture largely ill-prepared to cope with chronic pain. Understandably, he adds, patients feel the medical system has failed them.

A director of advocacy for patients with chronic pain has this to say: "For years I worked in a pain clinic. People who came to us had often gone to seventeen or eighteen other doctors before they came to us. They felt ignored, they felt angry, they felt sad, they felt frustrated, and they felt incredibly overwhelmed with grief and loss."[2] Says David Morris, "They shuttle from specialist to specialist, in a revolving door of referrals, seen so often by so many different doctors that finally no one really sees them."[3]

My situation exactly. A number of years into this trauma, after seeing physician number seventeen, I walked out of his office, feeling as if I were on a treadmill, going from doctor to doctor, feeling no one spent enough time with me to understand my problems. Twice I went to the wrong hospital, as hospitals and clinics blurred in my mind. The buildings all looked alike. The doctors all seemed to do the same thing. All checked my nerve responses. All asked me, "What happened?" and wrote down what I said. I have never understood why they have to repeat in their reports "what happened": "As you know, this pleasant lady had a motor vehicle accident in which she was broadsided..." Everyone already knows what happened from previous reports. Perhaps I may just say something that clicks in a doctor's mind in a way it has not for others, which could be a clue for a different treatment. So far that has happened only with my prolotherapist and my wellness physician (a physician who focuses on well-being, which can include an emphasis on nutrition, exercise, hormonal balance through the use of bio-identical hormones, meditation, relaxation, spirituality, and other alternative approaches to promoting health). Not because they heard something others had not but because they looked through different lenses themselves, listening to the same story with a different understanding of illness and healing.

To find professionals from among the many with alternative approaches who could bring about some temporary relief has been an equally difficult and confusing task that I essentially had to carry out myself. Only two of the many physicians and specialists I have seen suggested massage, acupuncture, or physiotherapy—the most commonly accepted alternatives. One other specialist sent me to an emotional release therapist, suggested I try magnets, and tested me for vitamin B-12, of which vegetarians (I have been a vegetarian for over thirty years) often do not have enough.

I have had anywhere from one to over thirty appointments with each of these sixty people. That is sixty different names and addresses to remember by an already exhausted and traumatized brain. To date I have had some 240 appointments with doctors and specialists, and nearly 500 appointments with alternative professionals. Add to that about a dozen appointments for tests and assessments. Many of these appointments were at clinics and hospitals an hour or more away from my home. I also attended a ten-day residential pain clinic. I have seen my prolotherapist in Vancouver thirteen times so far, requiring a full day of travel each time. Add countless hours spent making lists of questions for all these professionals, keeping track of prescriptions, bills, insurance correspondence, learning about chronic pain—all this on top of "managing" thousands of hours of pain, while your mind has gone mush and your memory keeps failing, and you have the picture of at least two full-time, demanding "jobs."

"What do you do all day?" asked a colleague who called me after hearing that I had to go on disability leave.

"I have pain. I manage pain. I see doctors," I said.

"Oh," she said. And after a brief pause she said, "But what do you *do* all day long?"

I have files on every doctor and write down my questions before appointments. I often ask the same question of several doctors when it concerns an important aspect of my problems. As my story will show, their responses have been, more often than not, contradictory. Maddening at times. I have walked out of their offices in utter confusion. What to believe now?

Virtually all references from the medical literature I cite note the lack of adequate training for general physicians in understanding and treating chronic pain and the difficulties of making chronic pain an integral part of the medical curriculum. Many doctors have had only a few hours of pain-management training, which for most translated into learning about drugs.[4] General practitioners may not even know the best specialist for a particular pain pattern, even if they are willing to refer you, which not all doctors are. I have had three family doctors since the accident. The first doctor did essentially nothing. He prescribed Toradol and told me "let's wait and see"—which turned out to be the worst possible advice. Well over half a year passed before he sent me to a neurologist, who flatly told me I'd be in pain all my life. My second family doctor also knew little but decided to run about twenty-five tests of all kinds to eliminate other possible reasons for pain and exhaustion. When they all came out fine, she sent me on to a good pain clinic. The third family doctor wanted to put me on morphine, but thankfully he was more than willing to refer me for prolotherapy when I asked him to, although he was not familiar with it. Indeed, I found knowledge of chronic pain, and the willingness to find out what can be done about it, to be very uneven among doctors. Says Scott Fishman, "Among doctors, treating patients in pain is widely viewed as one of health care's most challenging tasks because it calls on so many different areas of expertise. Most doctors today are not prepared to deal with this complexity, grounded as they are in single disciplines such as anesthesiology or neurology."[5]

Chronic pain patients need a coordinator, a guide, someone who understands both chronic pain and how the health-care system works—or doesn't work. Not to judge whether a doctor is right or wrong, but to keep track of the process, of what is happening with the patient. Someone who can prevent the patient from getting lost, confused, and feeling abandoned. Ostensibly, one's family doctor is supposed to do that, but often he or she lacks the required knowledge. People suffering from chronic pain need advocacy, says Arthur Rosenfeld.[6] But, he adds, unlike many other disabled people they cannot be their own advocates, as they don't have the required stamina or clarity of mind, disabled as they are by their constant pain. Many times I have felt I could not go another day advocating for myself. I would collapse for weeks. Then, somehow, I would force myself to focus and go at it again.

There are pain-management clinics, but still mostly only in the larger cities, and there aren't nearly enough of them. Wait time is often more than a year, sometimes even two or three years. Given that thousands of people walk around in serious and recurring pain, it is difficult to accept that not more doctors specialize in pain management. But there are reasons for that. The work is difficult. On October 16, 2005, Dr. Ellen Thompson, a pain specialist, told the *Ottawa Sun,* which ran a series of articles on chronic pain that month: "You burn out. It's very stressful. These are desperate people. We can only cure a few. We can ameliorate the situation for many, but there are a few that are intractable." Dr. David Corey, president of the interdisciplinary pain clinic of the Health and Recovery Group in Toronto, echoes the difficulty of the work in pain management. He told the *Ottawa Sun* on October 20, 2005, that patients who visit pain clinics can have their pain reduced to some degree. Their function improves and depression and anxiety become somewhat less severe. Statistically, these improvements range between 20 and 40 percent. Corey could only remember one case in twenty-five years in which the person had a complete elimination of pain. As a pain patient, I have to say that while these percentages of improvement are not high, they are significant for a life lived in pain. *Any* help is help.

Dr. Atul Gawande, in his book *Complications: A Surgeon's Notes on an Imperfect Science,* has this to say:

> Though we want to be neutral in our feelings toward patients, we'll admit among ourselves that chronic-pain patients are a source of frustration and annoyance: presenting a malady we can neither explain nor alleviate, they shake our claims to competence and authority. We're all too happy to have [a pain specialist] take these patients off our hands.[7]

Dr. Linda Wynne, anesthesiologist at the Ottawa Hospital Pain Clinic, told the *Ottawa Sun* on October 19, 2005, that the single largest problem they face is that many family doctors refuse to take patients back once they have attended the clinic. Marni Jackson says of doctors and their aversion to dealing with chronic pain, "If they can't fix it, they would prefer to fax it somewhere else."[8] Dr. Michael Stein, author of *The Lonely Patient,* admits that as a young doctor, he found his patients' pain to be unknowable; it felt far away, he says. He feared that if he came too close to pain it might cling to him. Patients who came to him over and over for pain relief at times bored him.[9]

To further confuse those in chronic pain, if you are lucky that there is a pain clinic where you live, and your doctor refers you to one, what will be offered depends on who runs the clinic. As pain specialists Doctors Mailis-Gagnon and Israelson have remarked, and as I found out, there are huge differences and disagreements among physicians with regard to what the correct approach is when it comes to chronic pain, and patients are often caught in the middle.[10]

The first time I was referred to a pain clinic I was still under the assumption that pain clinics are places where they can cure you. I have come to realize that many people think so. However, instead of cure, pain clinics offer "pain management." It essentially means: we will try to help you gain some level of control over your pain, but we cannot promise how much, or if we are going to be successful.

Listen to Your Doctor—and Buy Our Drugs

In the office of one of my doctors in Victoria is a very large poster on the door, titled "One Hundred Ways to Live to One Hundred." When you are waiting for him, you can't help reading it. Seven of the hundred ways are printed in bold as follows:

> Stop smoking; Exercise regularly; Reduce the amount of cholesterol in your diet; Take your medicine as prescribed; If you have had a heart attack or stroke and stopped taking your medication, speak to your doctor; Ask your doctor about new medication; Listen to your doctor.

In between, there are ninety three rules for longevity in normal print. The message suggests you can ignore them at no risk, while ignoring the boldly printed ones could be deadly. The fillers include such gems as: Eat your Brussels sprouts; Marry your sweetheart; Swim; Golf; Skinny dip; Look for rainbows; Bake a pie; Soak in the tub; Indulge yourself; Go fishing; Enjoy being single; Celebrate your marriage; Feed the birds. There are many more, but you get the idea.

The poster is the work of the pharmaceutical giant Bristol-Myers Squibb. I imagine recycled hippies along with the pharmaceutical-marketing staff quickly putting this poster together. Its basic message is simple: Listen to your doctor, who will prescribe for you the medications we sell. Add some of the most common sense health directives—stop smoking, reduce cholesterol, exercise—and there's your poster! Add to that the fact that pharmaceutical corporations fund huge amounts of medical research; provide funds for medical schools, medical conferences, patients groups, and for awards doctors receive; fund continuing medical education courses, setting the agenda for what doctors learn; and give doctors who prescribe their medicines gifts and cash and offer them various other incentives such as "all expense paid" workshops in exotic places, where they learn about the new medications the poster says you should ask your doctor about—and the extent of the pharmaceutical industries' influence on our health is clear.

Alan Cassels, a public health researcher, points out that doctors' claims that drug-marketing activity does not influence them flies in the face of what we know about marketing: in Canada alone, the pharmaceutical industry spends two billion dollars a year—which is $20,000 per doctor per year—on marketing to physicians.[11] I couldn't believe the figure and contacted him. "It's the correct figure," he said, "not a misprint." In the United States the industrywide marketing budget is estimated by researcher Marcia Angell at $54 billion, almost double the research-and-development outlays.[12] A former sales representative of a major pharmaceutical company told Gardiner Harris and Janet Roberts of the *New York Times* on March 21, 2007, "I hate to say it out loud, but it all comes down to ways to manipulate the doctors." Another one said, "The hope in all this is that a silent quid pro quo is created."

Becoming a chronic pain patient placed me right into this world.

The pharmaceutical infiltration into pain management narrows a doctor's understanding of pain and healing. This is the side of the story rarely asked: What is it that is *not* taught to doctors, as drug companies shape and narrow their education in so many ways? To date I have had twenty-three drugs tried out on me—many with major adverse effects and none bringing about permanent improvement. The most I get is some temporary relief in exchange for being made toxic. That I had to largely find out for myself about the various ways to ease pain without medication (addressed in chapter 5) is not unrelated to the impact the pharmaceutical industry has on what doctors learn—and don't learn. I would urge anyone to consider alternative approaches for pain relief along with drugs necessary to interrupt acute pain and dull severe pain. So far, alternative approaches have been the most helpful in strengthening my ligaments, straightening out and stabilizing my neck (thereby reducing inflammation, swelling, and pain), increasing endurance and energy, and keeping me somewhat sane. While drugs are of course necessary, and I continue to rely on them, alternatives are also needed because of the multiple modalities that interact with the brain in communicating about pain.

Listen to Your Doctor—but Which One?

In the sections to follow I tell of my interactions with my many health-care professionals. To provide a context for narrating these incidents I will first summarize the pain patterns I suffered from, the diagnoses I received, and the treatments that were provided. In recounting these incidents, I identify a medical professional as "physician" to indicate a family doctor and as "specialist" to indicate pain specialists, psychiatrists, neurologists, or surgeons. Each physician and each specialist within each category is a different person. Nonphysician health-care providers are identified by the nature of their professions. Only three physicians were female, and the great majority of the other health-care professionals were also male. To secure anonymity, I refer to everyone as "he."

Pain patterns: Swelling and pain in the neck and around the entire base of the skull, often spreading toward the top of my head; a large "glob" in my neck that swells and sets off what feels like electric shocks; headaches and full-blown migraines; referred pain in shoulders, upper back, and upper arms; facial pain around cheekbones and ears. These various pain patterns can flare up individually or all together. Over time, I started to experience exhaustion, depression, panic attacks, poor concentration, frequent nightmares, inability to tolerate noise, and severe sleep deprivation.

Diagnoses (overlapping in part): Closed head injury; whiplash; mechanical neck pain with facet joint trauma; displaced vertebrae; significant malalignment of the cervical vertebrae; loss-of-motion segment integrity at the C2 level indicative of a serious spinal condition; muscular ligamentous injury; unstable atlas bone; brainstem compression; cervical spondolysis; minor brain injury; traumatized cervical arthritis; occipital neuralgia; fibromyalgia; postconcussion syndrome; posttraumatic amnesia; myofascial syndrome; posttraumatic stress disorder; and major depression.

Treatments received: Drugs (anti-inflammatories, analgesics, anticonvulsants, opioids, antidepressants, muscle relaxants, lidocaine pain patches, Valium, sleeping pills); deep-tissue massage, acupuncture, osteopathic manipulations, chiropractic adjustments, intramuscular stimulation, and craniosacral and myofascial release work; a transcutaneous electrical nerve stimulation device (TENS); neural therapy (injections of lidocaine and anti-inflammatory substances into trigger points and other painful sites); rhizolysis (nerve cauterization) at levels C2 to C6, Botox injections, nerve blocks, and cortisone injections; prolotherapy; psychotherapy, emotional release therapy, and biofeedback; nutritional supplements and bioidentical hormone replacements. Treatments I initiated on my own have included mindfulness meditation, relaxation and deep breathing, and Tai Chi classes that focus on release of inner tension. I also took classes in the Alexander method, which teaches how to move so that no stress is exerted on the neck, and I am taking Iyengar yoga classes specifically designed for those with back and neck problems. In addition, I was advised by a neurosurgeon to have—but refused—open neck surgery to remove the nerve ganglion at the C1–2 level.

Had I tried to follow the often wildly differing and often contradictory advice of my many doctors I would have gone mad. Often I left a doctor's office, shaking my head, "What do I do now? Whom do I believe?" These many contradictions confronted me with the trial-and-error nature of pain management. But it also resulted from the fact that several doctors and specialists would only consider their own perspective and were ignorant, skeptical, or even disdainful of what others with different perspectives had to offer. The contradictions I encountered concerned almost every general diagnostic conclusion and treatment recommendation I would hear, including: the nature of the "glob" in my neck; the displacement of my vertebrae; the advisability, type, and need for exercise; use of traction; use of morphine; the correct placement of Botox injections; and the entire question as to whether or not I could get better.

General Diagnostic and Treatment Contradictions

Specialist: Traumatized arthritis. The nerves previously adjusted around arthritic bone spurs are now dislodged by the accident. They are irritated and give erratic messages to the muscles. "We see it all the time with car accidents," he said. Nothing can be done about it. I will be in great pain forever. He suggests massage and acupuncture for temporary relief.

Specialist: The nerves are overstimulated. Take a hot bath and rest for two hours each afternoon in absolute darkness. Take Celebrex at night. Go for as many massages as you can afford to keep the muscles soft. If I could manage, take a year's vacation and do absolutely nothing. He suggests a beach. I ask if he thinks the car insurance will pay for it. "Marry a rich man," is his creative solution. I called this "the Mexican beach theory." It is my favorite, but the Mexican beach never materialized.

Specialist: Facet joint damage that is not visible on an X-ray or MRI. The nerves at the damaged sites are irritated. We can burn your nerves where they exit the spinal canal.

Massage therapist: The vertebrae are out of place. The neck goes all zig-zag! No solution offered.

Specialist: Vertebrae out of place? That is not possible. They are very well-hooked together!

Specialist: There is a lot of instability in your neck.

Car insurance company: The MRI shows "nothing abnormal," therefore it appears that there is no "organic basis" for your continuing pain. Further claims are disallowed.

Massage therapist: Your muscles are overstretched. They need to be re-educated.

Craniosacral therapist: The myofascial tissue is much too tight and needs to be released.

Chiropractor: Given the facet joints are damaged, we need to adjust them back into place. (He tried by cracking my neck. It made the pain worse.)

Wellness physician: Because I was a vegetarian, I lacked the necessary protein to fight the constant inflammation and to build up weakened muscles. He advised protein supplements and bio-identical hormones.

Specialist: The force of the collision weakened the ligaments, which do not easily heal by themselves. Weak ligaments cause pain because they have nonstretchable nerve endings that hurt when under pressure from loose joints, and they also refer pain elsewhere. Treatments consist of injections into the ligaments every four to six weeks until they are strengthened and the neck is stabilized. His chiropractor colleague measured my atlas bone: it is off by three degrees, causing brainstem compression. Solution: computer-controlled gentle adjustments (no "cracking") along with the prolotherapy.

The Mystery of the "Glob"

I have asked a number of my doctors and specialists to tell me what this hard "thing" in my neck is and what can be done about it. This is what they told me:

Specialist: I ask him to feel my neck. I am not an expert in feeling necks, he says, coming from behind his desk. He feels the swelling. I don't know—could be a neuroma. I can send you to someone who can take it out.

Specialist: It's a neuroma. Never have it taken out. If you do, it will grow back, or you can get many little neuromas.

Specialist: It's not a neuroma—it's a bone. The bone is covered with sensitive nerves that are irritated. There is nothing to be done about it.

Specialist: This is *abnormal!* (Please God, not that.) Never felt anything like it! He immediately phones the neurosurgeon he had referred me to and with whom I just had had a consultation. It sounded, hearing only his side of the conversation, as if I could have a cancer or some other terrible condition. They decided to have another MRI done, which failed to show anything in that area.

Massage therapist: It is probably an entrapment of scar tissue and nerves. He works hard at massaging the entrapment into loosening up.

Massage therapist: It is a myofascial contraction. He too thinks massage is the answer.

Physician: It is not a neuroma or a myofascial problem. I think it's a swollen lymph node.

Specialist: It is a myofascial problem. The prolotherapy will loosen it little by little as the increasingly stronger ligaments will exert a steady pull on it.

Chiropractor: It does not matter what it is. It could be all of what you have been told. He tells me that what counts is to get my atlas and pelvis bones adjusted along with the prolotherapy and then the problem should disappear.

Chiropractor: You know what I think? It's brain fluid collecting in that area.

OK. Whatever. I collected these contradictory or partially contradictory diagnoses over a ten-year period. For me, this thing is now just a "glob." That is as good as it gets.

Dr. Jerome Groopman, chair of Medicine at Harvard Medical School, tells of a woman who developed chronic pain after she fell and hurt her knee.[13] These are the diagnoses she received from the first three orthopedic specialists: be patient, the wound will soon heal; cartilage fragments might have broken off the kneecap and lodged in the joint; I don't know, take opioids. A physiotherapist thought she probably had reflex sympathetic dystrophy (RSD). Still another orthopedic surgeon told her she did not have RSD, she had a neuroma. Another neurologist thought she had bone cancer, but a test showed no cancer and the neurologist changed his diagnosis to probably Lyme disease. That comes to seven different diagnoses for knee pain! Before my accident I would have thought this woman's experience was one of a kind. Now I know the world of chronic pain is characterized by such stories.

Exercise, Yes! Exercise, No!

The Canadian Back Institute: I am told to retract my neck, that is, to push my head back as far as possible and hold it there for a few seconds, and to do that ten times a day, as well as some related exercises—turning my head sideways as far as possible, and bending my ear to my shoulder.

A two-month generic physiotherapy program: We are told, over and over, that we have to come. Especially when in pain. At times the pain was so bad I was in tears. I would excuse myself and lie down in an adjacent room, but was asked to join again as soon as I possibly could.

Craniosacral therapist: He expressed horror at this: I should *not* do any exercises. First, my muscles have to heal. Only after healing would exercise be appropriate.

Physiotherapist: I must exercise. He prescribes some exercises similar to the physiotherapy program that brought me to tears. I also was told to use the "neck system" to strengthen my neck muscles. This is a flexible bar you put over the door. It has a small soft pad attached to the end. You put your head against the pad from various angles and push it toward the wall.

Massage therapist: I should follow the exercises outlined in *Take Care of Your Own Neck*. I buy the book and start doing the exercises, which are similar to those the Canadian Back Institute recommended.

Specialist to whom I show *Take Care of Your Own Neck:* Absolutely not. I have to be very careful. The only thing I am allowed to do is make tiny circles with my head to keep the center of my neck loose.

Specialist: No retraction exercises, as they compress the facet joints even further. He advises only gentle stretches having my head up and a bit forward.

Wellness physician: I need to exercise carefully. He shows me some beginning weight-lifting exercises with my arms, lifting them sideways and above my head.

Specialist: No exercising at all as long as we are doing prolotherapy.

The Ongley Pain Clinic in Ensenada, Mexico: This clinic specializes in prolotherapy (which they call "reconstructive therapy"). After injections, patients make small repetitive movements with their heads, sideways, and up and down, fifty times, twice a day. It is considered central to proper placement of new ligament fibers.

Specialist: No, don't do it. The normal day-to-day movements with your head takes care of that.

Traction, Yes! Traction, No!

Orthopedic physician: He tells me I have had every possible treatment. The only thing he can still recommend is a home traction kit that fits over a door. It consists of a trolley with a water bag on one side and a contraption made of cloth to put your head in at the other side. You adjust the water load in the bag to the prescribed weight, which pulls up your head to create space between the vertebrae.

Prolotherapist: Use it, but be very careful. You could hurt yourself.

Chiropractor: Do not use it. Absolutely not. It will create other problems.

Family doctor: If it at all makes you feel uncomfortable, I wouldn't use it.

Morphine, Yes! Morphine, No!

Anesthesiologist: He wanted me to be on morphine daily. There should be morphine in my system at all times. I tried it for two weeks but suffered such severe side effects that I had to stop.

Family doctor in Toronto: Take it only when absolutely needed (this is what I wanted to do).

Pain specialist in the Netherlands (horrified): We only give morphine to people who are terminally ill.

Family doctor and *pain specialist* in Victoria: Both wanted me to be on daily morphine again. I tried once more for three weeks. Side effects were again severe, particularly hallucinations and cognitive dissociation with a resulting inability to function.

Displaced Vertebrae, Yes. Displaced Vertebrae, Not Possible.

Initial X-rays taken in Toronto showed no vertebrae displacement. Two massage therapists, however, told me that several vertebrae felt out of place. A specialist told me that was not possible ("the vertebrae are very well-hooked together"). A subsequent computer analysis of the X-rays showed vertebrae subluxation at the C2 and C5 levels, as well as "loss of motion segment integrity at the C2 level in translation," referring to "an abnormal back-and-forth motion of one vertebra over another greater than 3.5 mm." Mine was 3.7 mm at the C2 level, which is indicative "of a serious spinal condition." I was told that just having this misalignment and loss of "motion segment integrity" could account for a large part of the pain I was experiencing. (This particular analysis was an important factor in my being granted a disability leave from work. It was *not* part of routine procedures, and I had to pay for it myself.) Three years later in Victoria, my prolotherapist and his chiropractor colleague also diagnosed major instability. By then, my neck was so unstable, so wobbly, that I often could *feel* the vertebrae shift.

Botox Here! No, There!

Pain specialist in Toronto: Injected Botox in the middle of my neck. Unfortunately, while it is helpful for many chronic pain sufferers, it did nothing for me. He told me I was one of those who immediately develop antibodies.

Pain specialist in Victoria: Tried Botox injections again, in the same place. Nothing happened.

Pain specialist in Vancouver: On hearing I had had Botox injections in the middle of my neck, he said, "Oh, no wonder. That is the wrong place! The injections need to go right where it hurts—here, and there!" He injected Botox in half a dozen places where the morning pain is most distinct. Nothing happened but a temporary adverse effect some people suffer from—a painful swelling in the areas injected.

*Prognosis: You Will Not Get Better; You May Get
Better; You Will Get Better*

Specialist: I have an elderly patient with your problems, and he can't turn his neck anymore without being in excruciating pain.

Physiotherapist: Three months and we will have you in good shape.

Physiotherapist (after I had had the nerve-burning procedure and was still having the same pain): Just have a good attitude. We will work on your neck, sow some seeds here and there, and when the nerves grow back they will be just fine, and your pain will be gone.

Physician: My problems are of a permanent incurable nature.

Specialist: Prognosis is poor. My condition tends to worsen over time.

Massage therapist: You have had this pain for seven years? Oh, then it will never go away.

Specialist: (I had expressed my despair at still being in pain when I am ninety.) No, don't think that way. Sometimes it just goes away. Why? I ask. We don't know why, he says. It burns itself out or something.

Specialist: There is no cure. Nothing can be done about it. He tells me to take morphine. I express my despair at still being in severe pain at the age of ninety. Not necessarily, he says. Sometimes it just goes away. Why? I ask. We don't know. Perhaps the bones get softer.

Prolotherapist and his *chiropractor colleague:* We can help you. But we do not know how much, given your injuries are serious and they have been there for so long.

To date, the prolotherapist and his chiropractor colleague have been closest to the truth. Improved, but not cured.

My Doctors: In how many ways do I know them?

The following vignettes recount my interactions with my doctors and specialists. Sixteen different medical professionals out of the twenty-two I have seen are represented. (My interactions with the other six didn't stand out one way or the other.) In how many ways have I come to know them? There are five: the fine ones; the "Do I have the cure for you!" ones; the bad-mannered ones; the science-obsessed ones; and the inappropriately cheerful ones.

The Fine Ones

Specialist: My favorite pain specialist in Toronto, Dr. Gordon Ko, has a healing touch. His hand rested often on my shoulder as he injected me with lidocaine, Sarapin (a plant extract that interferes with pain signals), or other natural or homeopathic anti-inflammatories. I often had to tell him how terrible the pain had been. He would say, "I am sorry" or "I know" followed by a kind pause. His demeanor always brought some peace to my soul. He was pleased to see me no matter how full his waiting room was. No matter that he knew he could not cure me. Dr. Ko was always very realistic and never made any promises, but he never gave up trying. He was the one who called me back at the end of the first visit and said, "Lous, one more thing, never give up." Though he put the ultimate responsibility for recovery on me, he was willing to try anything he could think of. He welcomed my questions. And he *did* bring about in these alternative approaches and, with his compassion and genuine kindness, some temporary relief.

Wellness physician: Dr. Charles Myers is a focused, friendly, straight-shooting man with a sense of humor. My first meeting with him was straightforward: he did a diet check, talked about exercise and a hormonal checkup, and then he spoke of psychological matters we would take up the next time. That made me nervous. I feared I would break down if I told him of my depression and despair. I hate it when I break down in front of doctors I do not like, as has happened more than once. A sense of pride is involved: that man is not going to see me break down. But then I don't want to break down in front of the ones I like either. In the end, however, I have no control over it. It depends on how much pain I am in. On whether I had any sleep. On whether I have had drugs that day that scramble my emotions. Or what questions the doctor asks. I am only consoled knowing that chronic pain patients often break down in their doctors' offices.

I decide to tell him of other difficulties. I want to keep it short and keep control of the story. I practice before I see him. I make note of the loss of my fine career. I mention the past half year in which a sister and a brother-in-law died, two of my cats died, another close relative developed cancer, I fell and sprained and re-sprained my ankle—and all of this while I was in increasing and often excruciating pain from my neck injuries. I mention the rhizolysis resulting in increased pain and nerve pain, which led to a three-year stretch of intense suicidal thoughts. He listens attentively. I am doing well and sticking with the outline I rehearsed in my mind. I am not falling apart. But I do not look at him when I mention the suicidal period. I tell him of the long, severe Toronto winters that made the pain worse and the isolation unbearable. I also point out I have had to move four times in five years.

"You have lost a life," he tells me. Finally, someone who got it. He tells me I registered at the far end of several stress scales. He is compassionate. I am refreshed because I sense he means it. It is one of the better medical appointments I have had. The scientific method was absent. He is not my psychotherapist, but as my doctor he also must have a sense of the state of my soul. There was no rush. We had an hour. His wellness counseling is a private practice. For the privileged ones. And that is of course the problem. When chronic pain is present, other difficulties weigh much more heavily. The fee-for-service system does not allow physicians to give patients with serious pain problems the time they need to get at some of the complexities of their lives that aggravate the pain.

Physician: The pain had started at home. I took a Tylenol 3 and felt I could make it to the doctor's office. But by the time I arrived the pain was in full swing. My neck muscles were in a painful spasm, and the base of my neck was so weak I thought my head would fall off. I could not sit on the small chair in his office and instead paced in front of him, holding my neck in both my hands, my eyes tearing. He had nothing to offer, and I felt badly for him. I had stepped to the side in a failed attempt to keep my composure, to not have to look in his eyes. "I know you don't have the answers either," I said. He quietly responded, "But I can listen." Immediately, I experienced a certain calmness. I felt relieved. Here was a doctor acknowledging that, indeed, he did not have the answer either. But he spoke truth. He would listen. And he did.

I asked him to refer me to Dr. Nasif Yasin for prolotherapy. He had never heard of prolotherapy but was immediately interested. I brought him Ross Hauser's book on prolotherapy. Looking through it, he said, "This is exciting for me too." He went on, "Perhaps I should learn how to do that. There must be places where they train you." To be so open about his lack of knowledge was a key to my trust in him—a doctor who had no problem exposing the limits of his knowledge, welcoming what I brought him.

Specialist: Dr. Nasif Yasin, with a handshake and a warm welcoming smile, said, "Ah, you are Gordon Ko's patient. We went to school together!" His accent told me he was not from North America. Later on, as I lay on the table and he took a break from putting needles into me, I asked where he was from. He was born in Libya. Having grown up in the Netherlands, and having lived for several years in South America where personal interactions are warmer and more relaxed, I have often been struck by how distant and businesslike many North American medical professionals can be. I was going to like this doctor. It would be a pleasure to visit him even though he would be putting painful needles into my neck.

Impeccably dressed in suit and tie, Dr. Yasin sits down and faces me with an open and direct look. He asks very detailed questions. Did I have my foot on the pedal when the accident happened? Exactly how fast were the cars going? Was I looking straight ahead or to the side? No other doctor had asked such precise questions. He listens attentively, nodding, taking notes. "OK, let's hop on to the table and let me feel your neck." Finally, after more than six years of assessments, tests, and more assessments, a miracle happens: Someone *carefully feels my neck!*

This is entirely new. Previous medical appointments consisted mainly of verbal exchanges. Doctors who felt my neck did so quickly. Some never felt my neck. Their initial diagnoses were based on information I provided or on reports they had been given. In follow-up appointments they relied on their own formal test results. But this Dr. Yasin used his hands as a diagnostic tool. The displacement of the neck vertebrae that initial X-rays had not picked up on he felt immediately.

He works his way slowly and carefully down my neck, talking to himself, as if to make sure he will remember it all. I catch a few phrases: "C1 is here...C2 should be there...a subluxation..." and much more I do not understand. His fingers, firm yet gentle, slowly move from one vertebra to the next, feeling their way though all the bends and curves. His words go right along with his fingers. I felt excitement, lying on my stomach, my view restricted to his shiny beige shoes. This man knows my problems.

He began his treatment with a series of local anesthetic injections just under the skin, followed by perhaps a dozen much deeper injections with dextrose into the ligaments. I was breathing in and out slowly and deeply to relax as much as possible. He guided me through it verbally, yet was firm in his movements, putting the needles into my neck and working them around muscles and other tissues to the spot where the ligaments attach to the bone. He would stop in between injections, let his arm fall down his body to rest, and ask, "How are you doing?" and wait for me to answer. Nothing was rushed. While it was no picnic, it was not all that bad either. The injections hurt less than the nerve blocks I had had and cortisone injections I would have later on. In fact, they became progressively less painful over the course of the treatments.

At the end, he administered a series of small anesthetic injections all around my skull, including my forehead, and said gently, "This will make you sleep well tonight."

A doctor who cared about how I would sleep! In the initial conversation I started to cry when he asked how I was sleeping. "Sleeping," I said, "for years..." and I broke down. I wanted to tell him I had not had a single night of normal sleep for years. But I couldn't finish my sentence. My daughter who was with me took over. "Her whole life has been taken away," she said, as if to explain my breaking down. Through my tears, I felt the doctor's eyes resting kindly on me. His demeanor was consistent with what was to follow: empathetic, quiet for a few moments, then gently proceeding with his questions.

After he was done with the injections, I got up and said, "Wow, it felt as if an artist was feeling my neck!"

"Ah... the beauty of it!" he exclaimed. My daughter had been watching. She told me later he had seemed like a concert pianist. Totally concentrated, intensely focused, a performance of artistic mastery. We left his office, feeling we had found the best possible answer to my problems so far.

Physician: My current family doctor, a complementary physician, is never rushed, often gives me a bit more time, and badly wants to help me. A friendly yet to-the-point doctor who speaks in a kind tone, he is always open to whatever questions I have, big or small. He looks over information I gather from the Internet that I have questions about. I go to him both before I have an appointment with a specialist, to help me to think through what questions I need to ask, and after I have seen the specialist, to talk over what transpired and so I can get his views. It is great to have a doctor who is willing to serve as an adviser. Just recently, after I had to tell him that another medication he wanted me to try out had done nothing for the pain, he gestured despair with his hands and said, "I'm just groping." Feeling badly for him, as well as affection—he so much wants to help me—I told him that I *really* did not expect him to cure me. That I was very happy I could come to him without being nervous, always feeling I could ask him any question. And I thanked him for not giving up on me, for never showing any sign of impatience. I trust he believed me.

The "Do I have the cure for you!" Ones

I asked the ER doctor who first examined me in the small Ontario rural hospital when he thought I could go home.

"Tomorrow," he said. "We'll keep you overnight just in case."

"Tomorrow?" "How will I get home? My car is totaled! It is a two-hour drive!"

"You can rent a car." Then, retreating somewhat he said, "That may not be a good idea right after an accident."

"No, I think not," I responded in disbelief. A few minutes later I asked, "When do you think I can go back to work?"

"Oh, in about two weeks." The next morning he bent over me and remarked, "You are quite a sight!" A nurse helped me to the bathroom where I looked in the mirror. My eyes were hidden in black-and-blue tissue. The upper half of my face was completely swollen. My body hurt so bad that I could not sit or walk unaided. A test showed blood in my urine. I had terrible headaches. Driving home in a rental car the next day? Going back to work in two weeks?

Physiotherapist: "Three months and we'll have you in good shape." This was almost three years after the accident. He had done the usual things: a hot towel under my neck, minor neck massage, and then sent me to the exercise room. I asked what he thought of my chances for improvement. "Three months." It was the first time that I immediately mistrusted a professional. By then I knew that three months of what he offered was not going to do it. Since then, I have listened carefully to what health professionals tell me with a sense of critical detachment.

Chiropractor: He had me stand up to judge my posture, and then he felt my neck: "I think I can help you. I have an 80 percent success rate with my clients." "Really?" I said. Still hoping, of course, though now with doubt lodged in my mind. I let him crack my back and my neck. It made things worse. I went back and had it done again. It made it worse. I decided I would not be among the 80 percent of patients he was successful with.

Specialist: He advised doing a rhizolysis.

"A rhizolysis, does that mean no more pain?" I asked.

"Yes, that's what it means, at least not until the nerves grow back."

"When will that be?"

"The average is about eleven months."

"Can you do it again then?"

"Oh, yes, we can do it again. You do have to count on about five days to recuperate. There'll be some pain."

"So, the solution is burning my nerves about every year and I can be free of pain?" I hardly believed what I had heard. Hope again! He nodded. I was elated. The nightmare would soon be over. I was so excited it didn't even occur to me that no mention had been made of possible adverse effects. I went ahead and scheduled the tests that had to be done first to make sure that it was indeed my facet joints that caused the problem.

The tests were extraordinarily painful, something I had not been told. During the testing procedure, instead of burning the nerves, a freezing substance is injected at the site where the nerves are to be burned to make sure that the pain stops when the nerves are rendered dysfunctional. Two nurses were also in the operating room. One, it turned out, was mainly there to hold my hand. She knew it was going to be tough. The surgeon had to do it at five levels. On two different occasions. Lying there waiting for the next needle to go in, I did not know if I could go on with it and I said so. His response: "Some people can't."

"What do you do then?"

"We stop." He went on to say when that happens the rhizolysis cannot proceed. He failed to tell me how painful the tests were going to be, possibly out of fear I might opt out. I understood his worry but felt a bit betrayed. The terrible surprise seemed very unfair.

The rhizolysis was done in a Toronto hospital. The procedure is painless, thanks to intravenous pain killers, which cannot be given during the tests as the patient has to be able to give feedback. Rather than having five days of pain, hell followed and lasted for almost two months. First, there was increased pain everywhere. Second, there was a spot, just above where one of the needles had gone in and the size of a large coin, where I developed nerve pain: a terrible burning and stinging pain, so bad, that I could not touch it. I could not comb my hair. I could not lie either on my left side or on my back. In both positions the spot touching the pillow caused unbearable pain. I sat up nearly day and night in the La-Z-Boy.

I called the specialist who had done the procedure. He understood my experience immediately and finished my attempts to describe the pain. "You can't comb your hair, you can't touch it—that's nerve pain," he said. "Didn't I tell you that could happen?"

"No, you didn't."

He apologized. "I must have forgotten. It happens to 4 percent of patients. It will go away in about six weeks," he said.

"Are you sure," I asked in despair, not believing any doctor on his word anymore.

"I am sure."

"What about the increased pain everywhere else?" I asked.

"That happens to 5 percent of people. Didn't I tell you that?"

"No, you didn't tell me that either," I said. What else had he not told me?

"Didn't my receptionist give you a handout with all the facts on it?" he asked. No, she had not. I received the handout at the follow-up appointment. But should possible risks be conveyed on a handout given by a receptionist? As a patient, I needed to be able to ask questions. Risks should be discussed, not just listed on a piece of paper.

I do not know how, for almost two long months, I lived with constant and furious pain, from hour to hour. Drugged out of my mind. It is a dark, dark spot in my memory. I became seriously suicidal. Detailed plans. Only the thought of my daughters stood between me and death.

Then, the nerve pain—which does not respond well to pain medications—softened and almost disappeared. The pain that had been on the left side of the neck improved, but only to make room for sharp pain two inches toward the middle of the neck. I have since learned such operative procedures often simply shift the pain symptoms elsewhere. Chronic pain, says David Morris, seems to follow a complex network of crisscrossing highways. If you cut off the interstate route, the pain impulse will frequently take to the back roads.[14] On balance, after the two horrendous months of increased pain and added nerve pain was over, there was some 20 percent improvement compared to before the rhizolysis. Then, six months later, the pain crept back up to where it had been before. How could this be?

On the handout from the secretary I learned that "complete pain relief is not to be expected." Fifty to eighty percent relief is considered successful. It also mentioned that the procedure is successful by this definition for only 60–65 percent of pain sufferers. The referring doctor never told me about success rates, though he mentioned it in his report to the insurance agent later on, a copy of which I obtained. Nor did he spell out for me what "successful" meant. He led me to believe it would work. That it always worked. Here I was. Back to square one.

Specialist: He took extensive notes and asked a lot of questions. Since the rhizolysis had not worked, he was to consider a C2 ganglion open neck surgery. He examined me and said I was a good candidate for the operation. I asked how many he had done. About a hundred, he said with some pride. I would be in the hospital for five days. After the operation there would be a lot of pain for a few days, after which the pain would disappear. "Altogether?" I asked. He nodded. A cure! There was a cure after all. I should think it over and, if I decided to go ahead, call for an appointment with still another doctor for another assessment where—just as with the tests for the rhizolysis—they would freeze the place in my neck where they would operate to see if that would indeed take the pain away.

I asked about side effects. What could go wrong?

"Nothing, really," he answered.

"Could I develop nerve pain afterward?" Note that *I* had to ask the question. He had not said a word about possible adverse effects, though I had told him I had developed nerve pain from the rhizolysis.

"A small possibility," he said, "about 5 percent of people do."

Rather than reassurance, I felt fear creeping up my spine. "If that happens," I asked, "what can you do about it?"

"Nothing," he said bluntly. Then he added, "Marijuana might help. I just spoke this morning with the wife of one of my patients who had the operation. He developed nerve pain, and marijuana is helping." The casual tone in which all this was said made me angry.

"Given I did develop nerve pain after the rhizolysis, would my chances therefore be higher than 5 percent for your operation?"

"Possibly," he said "but not necessarily." Perhaps that is indeed all he could say. But why had he not told me of these possible adverse effects up front?

Then and there I decided not to put my fate in this man's hands. I could see myself sitting straight up in my easy chair for hours on end, smoking pot for nerve pain for the rest of my life. I checked with my pain specialist, the referring doctor, the anesthesiologist who had done the rhizolysis, and with my family doctor. All said, "Don't do it." All saw the operation as a very last resort. The anesthesiologist literally said, "I can tell you this. If you were to develop nerve pain from that operation, it will be much worse than what you had after the rhizolysis. It will never go away and no one could do anything about it." How is it possible that a surgeon seriously suggested this operation, with no mention of these risks?

The Bad-Mannered Ones

Specialist: This was my second appointment with the first specialist I ever saw. The first time, almost a year after the accident, he had done all the neurological testing. Knowing I taught in the faculty of education at York University, he spoke of his young son in first grade and how his son's teacher went about teaching in the wrong way. What would I do if I were he? As I lay there enduring the needles, he chatted on about his own life. The second appointment lasted just a few minutes. I was told I had "traumatized arthritis." "Nature is kind," he said. When osteoarthritis forms, the nerves adjust themselves around the bone spurs. But my accident had dislocated them from their adjusted position and now they no longer knew how to go back. They were now sending erratic messages to my muscles: hence the muscle spasms I was experiencing.

"What can you do about it?" I asked eagerly.

"Nothing can be done about it," he said matter-of-factly. "Just make sure you don't have another accident. Don't fall. Don't walk on uneven ground." The latter I could do, but how could I control the other things? I was beginning to get the first intimations of what lay ahead.

"What kind of prognosis do you have for me?" I asked.

He never looked up as he answered; instead, he kept his eyes on my file. "I have an elderly patient with your problems. He is in a wheel chair and cannot turn his head anymore without being in excruciating pain." These were the exact words of his reply. They are inscribed in my mind. Forever.

"Is that what I have to look forward to?" I felt as if lightening had struck me.

He seemed to realize what he had just said and pulled back a bit. "We'll have to see, time will tell."

I don't remember how I got out of there. In tears, I drove immediately to my family doctor, who was kind enough to work me in. He calmed me down. "Let's not necessarily believe that," he said.

"You think I can get better?"

"That is always possible," he said. Though he himself never did anything to contribute to that possibility.

Psychiatrist: It is October 2001. Toward the end of our first appointment, he puts an appointment card in front of me, date and time already filled out, and says: "I'll see you in a month." I was already put off by his arrogant demeanor during the interview. This was it.

"I don't understand why you need to see me again," I said.

"I see my patients every month."

"I was sent here for you to order an MRI." He looked at me and said, "You are depressed." Of course I was depressed. But I was referred to him not because I needed psychiatric treatment but, I had been told, because he could order an MRI faster than the pain clinic could.

He had asked me a series of questions from a list. Are you depressed? Do you think of death? Are you unhappy? Of course I hit them all. I broke down a bit when all these questions were fired at me, and I tried to answer them honestly. He wrote something on his prescription pad and put it in front of me, "I am putting you on Prozac." Not, what do you do about your depression? Not, what would you think of taking an antidepressant? An order instead.

"I don't think so," I said, as matter-of-factly as I could.

"Why not? Don't you want to feel better?" he asked, surprise in his voice.

"Yes, but not with Prozac," I said, pushing the prescription back toward him.

"Why not?" His voice was argumentative.

"I think it is normal to be depressed about all this pain, don't you?" I asked. No answer. "I deal with this depression differently." I let it hang. Giving him a chance to ask what I did about feeling depressed. As I recall, he just shrugged his shoulders. I did not feel like explaining to this man what I did to deal with my depression. His questions were abstract and did not deal directly with my life in chronic pain. To him, it did not seem to matter much what I was depressed *about*. We never went into any of the details of my life in pain. His entire performance had an abstract and routinized quality to it, something he did many times a day. How often, I wondered, did he routinely prescribe Prozac to people who said "yes" to a set number of questions on his list?

Signaling the end of the meeting, he handed me the appointment card with a date and time already on it. Another order. I knew I could make it, but I was not going to play on his terms. "I don't have my diary with me. I'll check and call you back." Right then and there I decided I would come back only to get the MRI results and this patriarchical doctor would not see me again.

Specialist: I had been in the waiting room for half an hour when he called me into his office. I had come to hear the results of tests. I sat down. He was busying himself at the fax machine. "This will take a few minutes," he said. He was waiting for several pages to come through and then started to read them. I figured the fax had to be my test results and he needed to first read through them. Why otherwise would he keep me sitting there, already a half hour behind and with others waiting in his waiting room?

"Those are my reports?" I asked naively.

"Oh, no," he said, "they've renewed my grant! Good news!" Meanwhile I was sitting there in pain, waiting for test results that could either be good or bad news for me. Apparently, my time was immaterial, his grants more important than my pain.

Specialist: The young resident called me in. I had traveled to a large teaching hospital in Toronto where I was to see a well-known surgeon for a second opinion about a possible ganglionectomy, or for any other advice he might have. It was bitterly cold, and it had taken me over an hour to get there. I was in mild pain leaving the house, but it slowly had gotten worse.

The young resident did all the preliminaries. I told my story for the umpteenth time. He left, and a few minutes later the distinguished-looking graying surgeon came in with the young resident in tow. He asked for more details. Then, he walked over to me and without warning screwed my neck. In the manner one unscrews a medicine bottle: pushing down forcefully on the crown and turning my head all the way sideways, much further than it could go by itself, in both directions. The pain was excruciating. My body jerked and I moaned. Then it was over. "Sorry I had to hurt you," he said. It sounded like a statement that came with his job requirement.

No one, *ever*, had done that. I felt completely violated. Those few who have examined my neck went about it carefully and warned me if they had to push somewhere in a manner that might hurt. I knew I was the object of a demonstration. While he had said nothing to me, he was talking to the resident. And what a lesson this resident was learning: hurt a patient without warning—all you have to say afterward is "sorry, I had to hurt you."

I also knew I would go into a major pain attack within minutes. No one could manipulate my neck as he had without causing a pain attack. All I could think of was how would I get home.

He crossed his legs. He told me that he did not think open neck surgery was the answer. "Do you have pain every day?"

"Oh, yes."

Looking at me with soft grandfatherly eyes he said, "I really feel for you." Then, almost as if talking to himself he added, "How a moment of inattention can ruin a life."

A ruined life? *What* did he say? He had just written off my future. I had been working so hard not to let that possible truth dictate my emotions. Who was this man? I remember his eyes soft with pity. It struck me that he was thinking of himself, what if *he* were to be damned to a life of pain? His life would be ruined. He would no longer be able to be a distinguished-looking surgeon. He made no attempt in the few minutes he had to tell me about my ruined life, to say anything that might have given me some hope, some healing. I don't know how I walked out of that office. I don't know if I said good-bye. I hope I didn't.

The pain exploded within minutes, just before I found the door to the street. My head was pounding. I walked on blindly. I could not find the subway. I knew that I could not drive home. Gunshots were going off in my head. My neck and shoulder muscles turned to steel. In tears, I walked and walked, the freezing wind blowing in my face. Finally, I recognized where I was. I needed to lie down. I struggled onto the subway and got out at Bloor Street, where I knew there was a·small movie theater where I could lie down in the darkness. At this time of day it would not be crowded. I picked an Italian movie. I went to the washroom and took two more Tylenol 3s and two Toradols. There were only a handful of people in the theater. There was just enough space behind the last row and the back wall. No one saw me. Not that I cared at that point. Using my coat as a pillow, I collapsed on the floor in intense pain and intensely alone. The melodious sound of the Italian dialogue was soothing. The pills started to work, and I fell into a deep kind of rest, a dulled version of the pain hovering over me, persistent in its presence.

When the movie ended, I felt strong enough to take the subway again and then drive home. I made a point of telling my referring pain specialist about my experience. "I'm not asking you to do anything about it," I said, "but I do want you to know what this man did." He seemed taken aback, just looked at me, but he said nothing.

Physician: He gave me a survey at the end of my appointment as I was about to leave, saying, "Would you be so kind as to fill it out?" The survey threw a forced choice question at me: Did the cream help the pain, "yes" or "no?" The doctor had put some antipain cream on my neck at the be-ginning of the appointment. I was taken aback and told him I could not answer the question with a clear "yes" or "no." We had been talking about various matters, which had distracted me from the low-level pain I had come in with. Moreover, when the pain level is low, it often comes and goes within minutes. He knew that about me. "Oh, another research project," I said, knowing he was involved in several of them. He smiled. "No, I can't fill it out," I said. I told him that neither a "yes" nor a "no" answer would be ac-curate. Happily, he did not push me. It reinforced, however, my suspicion of so-called research findings unless careful descriptions are provided of the conditions under which the research was carried out.

Physician: Also at the end of my appointment, he gave me a question-naire, asking among other things whether my visits to the clinic had less-ened the pain, had given me more energy—and the rest I do not know because I stopped reading. I knew at once I could not fill anything out. He needed testimonials, he said, to promote the work they were doing at the clinic. I told him it was far too early in the process for me to assess the results. We were not done with the treatments, and, as he knew, I was still having plenty of pain. "I know this would not be an accurate response," I told him. He agreed that it probably was too early for me to say anything definite about the effect of the treatments.

Having worked in social science all my professional life, I know my answers would have been used, not to get at truth, but to claim truth—quite a different matter. How many patients, I wonder, knowing nothing of proper research methods, when handed a questionnaire at the end of an appointment, would say, "Hey, wait a minute, this isn't the right time to ask me this. I can't answer that question." Even with my background in research design, I had a hard time doing so.

The Science-Obsessed Ones

Physician: Several years before the accident I was diagnosed with severe osteoarthritis in my thumbs (now nicely healed by prolotherapy) and was given anti-inflammatories, but the pain kept getting worse. I was told I could have cortisone injections only once or twice, because cortisone can make things worse in the long run. I had to wear hard splints at night and soft ones during the day.

Around that same time I read about glucosamine and decided to try it. As promised by the literature, after about two to three months, there was substantial improvement. While the pain was not entirely gone, I could now live with it. I was greatly relieved and mentioned it to my doctor.

"Oh, yes, glucosamine," he said.

"You knew about it?" I asked, incredulously.

"Yes, but there are no scientific studies on it," he said.

"It has been used for a long time, and there are thousands of people for whom it works!"

"But there are no double-blind studies on it," he said again.

"Can it harm me?" I asked, thinking that adverse effects might be the reason he had not mentioned it.

"Oh no," he said, "it is just a nutritional supplement."

Let me see if I get this right. No harmful side effects at all, thousands of testimonials, but no double-blind studies, therefore: No good. He would have agreed to cortisone shots. There were double-blind studies—probably lots of them—showing that cortisone, a strong anti-inflammatory, will take the pain away. Unfortunately, it can eventually make things worse as it eats away at whatever cartilage is left. But at least we have double-blind studies. That means *we can explain* that cortisone shots are the cause of the temporary improvement. Thus, the only reason glucosamine was not offered as a treatment by this doctor, no matter its long history of clinical success, was that the scientific method had not been applied to it. The only reason cortisone was acceptable, no matter it's long-term serious adverse effects, was that the scientific method had been applied. Doctors could be sure that cortisone was indeed the agent that brought about the effect. They could explain why it worked. *They* could explain. I suddenly saw, crystal clear, how it plays itself out when a doctor's primary goal is to act according to the scientific training he or she has received, and how that can be to the detriment of the patient. Why didn't this doctor say, "You can try glucosamine. There's no scientific evidence it works, but many people swear by it and it can't hurt." What could be more simple?

Specialist: My pain specialist referred me to a marijuana specialist to see if that might be the way for me to go. I told my anesthesiologist. He was visibly upset I was even considering it. "I can explain to a group of doctors exactly how Tylenol works, but no one knows how marijuana works!" he said with some agitation. With this doctor, too, the most important matter was, not to try everything possible to relieve my pain, but to do only that which he could explain. This doctor also became upset when I mentioned someone else had suggested trying magnets. "I know nothing about magnets," he said with obvious disdain. I learned later, that no one knows exactly how magnets work, but they do help some people. He also believed any and all manipulations were of no use.

To believe that drugs and operations are the only proper approaches, because they have a science behind them that the doctor can explain, is at odds with the complex, shifting, and interactive nature of chronic pain, involving as it does mind, body, spirit, and the day-to-day conditions of one's life. On the one hand, medical science has performed brilliantly. On the other hand, it also has denied and ignored much, which can be to the detriment of the patient.

The Inappropriately Cheerful Ones

Specialist: His self-congratulatory cheerfulness found its ultimate expression when he said, "Now we have isolated the source of the problem at the C1 level. That is significant!" For a moment I thought he had said something I should be happy about. But a split moment later it hit me: he was cheerful about *his* skills, about having diagnosed my problems correctly. I suddenly felt a spectator. This wasn't about me. It was about him. He decided that the C1 level, which he called an "exquisitely sensitive joint," was the main culprit. Since nothing can be done at that level, as it is too close to a major artery, he sent me home, telling me to learn to live with it and take morphine.

Specialist: The three times I had to see this man, he never had more than a few minutes for me. This time I saw him to discuss assessment results. He did all the talking, and I had no chance to ask any questions. He put up an X-ray of my back and said enthusiastically, "No wonder you also have back pain. Look here! There is a substantial scoliosis [curvature of the spine]. Right here!" He seemed to be happy about his diagnosis. I just sat there. No treatment was suggested.

Specialist: During the winter of 2006, the pain got suddenly worse again and my doctor referred me to still another specialist, the one who injected Botox in the places where it hurt.

"How did it go?" he asked at a follow-up visit. I had slept three hours that night, waking up to intense pain. I was exhausted. I told him there had been no pain relief—instead I had developed painful swelling for about two weeks. Sudden tears appeared and for a moment I couldn't speak. He looked at me for a second, lowered his eyes to my file and said, in an uplifting, soothing, almost cheerful voice, "Don't worry, dear. Don't worry. Let's not worry."

These silly words at once threw me back into focus, and I said, "How can I *not* worry after ten years of this, when there is nothing else you can do!" He looked at me for a brief second but said nothing. I felt spoken to as if I were a child who had scraped her knee from a bad fall. What goes on in the mind and emotions of a doctor who speaks that way?

Perhaps doctors' cheerfulness while the news is bad serves as a cover-up for their own disappointment that they cannot help you, or for what they perceive as the limitations of their knowledge. But that limitation is only real within a model of medicine that draws its boundaries tightly and in which only specialized knowledge is valued.

It has not been pleasant recalling these hurtful interactions with physicians. Similar incidents, however, also show up in tales related by other chronic pain patients. The damaging effects of such interactions are serious: they increase patients' suffering and alienation, and diminish hope and the courage to relay crucial information to one's physicians. These damaging effects are real and need to be acknowledged in medical education and in the medical literature.

The Patient-Doctor Interaction:
For Better or Worse

Since for many of us chronic pain remains resistant to treatment, the patient-doctor relationship is both crucial and demanding. As Nellie Radomsky observes, "Doctors and patients have minimal difficulty with acute pain problems. If you've broken your leg, sprained your ankle, developed appendicitis…quite likely you can find doctors who listen and act quickly. But now [with chronic pain] the story is different."[15] Chronic pain, says David Morris, is as different from acute pain as cancer is from the common cold.[16] It requires a entirely different doctor-patient relationship.

Visits to my bad-mannered, science-obsessed, or inappropriately cheerful doctors are nerve-racking. Afterward, I am often back on the street, confused, with another drug prescription in my hand, but none of my questions answered. Or, I received an answer but don't remember it, for the explanation was too short and too fast. How can it be that going to visit a doctor increases my pain?

The fine ones are another story. My time with them, however short, is quality time. They have become an extended family of sorts. Given that the life of a person living with serious pain problems is thin on social relations, appointments with fine doctors serve a relational, as well as a medical, function. My forced solitude and isolation is broken when there is someone who really wants to hear how I am doing. Someone I can freely talk to about the overriding factor in my life.

A good doctor-patient relationship, says Philip Coulter, serves a therapeutic function, "something well-observed elsewhere, but nowhere more so than in pain management."[17] Pain specialist Dr. Angela Mailis-Gagnon agrees:

> We teach our students the biomedical model. We teach them to be exceptional scientists and physicians…but we don't teach them that well to use

the greatest healing tool we have in our hands, and that is the personal—the mind, the soul, the heart—and how much we can mobilize in a successful relationship between [the doctor and patient]…not only from the emotional point of view, but from the neurophysiological point of view and what it does to your body and what systems it activates and what neurotransmitters are within you to make this happen.[18]

My appointments with my doctors directly affect my emotions, my neurophysiology, my neurotransmitters—all of which, for better or worse, have an impact on my pain.

Doctors who do not develop their personal power will remain half-doctors, says Eric Cassell.[19] True healing power, he says, operates apart from the technology and comes from within the physician. The antithesis of healing, he adds, therefore can also take place. There is no doubt in my mind that my bad-mannered, rushed, science-blinded, and inappropriately cheerful doctors have made my pain worse. Their projected neutrality points not to an absence of actual relationship but to a denial of one. I am not saying these doctors do not care. The nature of their caring, however, is constrained by what they see as their primary focus—listening to my words in order to process them into the scientific categories that they hold in their minds. They are not present. It is a form of caring that leaves out the human being. "We deny that this distancing is a choice," says Dr. Michael Stein.[20] The need to distance is presented in medical school as a necessary rule, he says, as a requirement of composure. It wasn't until his own brother became very ill that Stein realized that he did not have a vocabulary of illness with which to speak even to his own brother.

"How has your pain been?" my family doctor asks. This is during the worst years. It is a question I can no longer answer, for the pain has become indistinguishable from the rest of a life that is no longer a life. I want to say I am terrible. I can't take the pain anymore. I want to end my life.

Instead I say, "Up and down. Today the pain is bad. Last week I had a few decent days." I try to give an answer that he can handle within the few minutes we have. It is a strange feeling—wanting to protect my doctor from the chaos and pain of my life. Not because I don't think there is no need for him to know; I emphatically think there is. But the way the system is organized doesn't allow for that to occur. A young woman in severe chronic pain told me, "I smile and say, 'I am fine.' Why do I do that? I hate it when I do that. I am not fine. I am terrible. But I tell him that I am fine. I don't know why I am afraid to tell the doctors the truth." And a woman, herself a physician, suffering from chronic pain told me, "Why is it I tell my doctor I'm having a few good days but I don't tell him that the three previous weeks were terrible?"

Not telling doctors the truth may be in part because we fear the doctor will not really believe us anyway, for how can we convincingly tell of this pain they can neither see nor measure? In part it may be for our own psychological and cultural reasons—the need to hold oneself together, not wanting to complain. But it is also a result of having to deal with doctors whose mind-sets are shaped by the distancing ideology of science and of having to count the minutes.

My fine doctors heal by their kindness, grace, their genuine regret that they can't cure me, by touch, attentiveness, their welcoming of dialogue—even by their gentle sense of humor. Such healing messages contribute to a patient's well-being, soften pain, and foster the energy needed to "never give up." Between visits you know that you have someone who cares, who will help in any way he or she can. You feel no tension, no increase in pain before an appointment. No question is seen as unimportant. You look forward to the next visit, though you know he or she will not have the cure for you. That is the gift of healing. I adore my fine doctors. I do not know how they do it—day in, day out—with people like me.

Listening is never "just" listening. Not a waste of a doctor's time. Given that mind, body, emotions, the nervous system, neurotransmitters, and whatever else makes up a human being are intimately intertwined in the chronic pain experience, a doctor's attentive listening is medicine—in a supreme sense of the word. Eric Cassell cites studies showing that most medical students are not sure if relief of suffering is part of their work.[21] Cassell's writings are an eloquent plea to recognize that it is. The basic goal or relieving suffering, he says, is to restore the intactness of the person, and caring listening is the major avenue to bringing this about. Assigning the task for listening to a psychiatrist, says Cassell, may serve other functions, but it does not replace the patient's need to speak to the doctor caring for the illness. As a pain patient, I do not need my doctor to be my psychotherapist. However, a genuine attentiveness to my problems, a sense of empathy for what I am going through, a readiness to *hear* me—the things that my few fine doctors do for me—is that too much to ask for?

I relate to Dr. Gawande's reaction to a display case in a pain clinic that contained letters by patients to their pain specialists.[22] These letters were not quite the typical testimonials that doctors like to put up, Gawande comments. These patients did not thank the doctors for a cure. They thanked them for taking their pain seriously—for believing in it. With my few fine doctors, I have never experienced a sign of disbelief, a lack of patience, a being bored with my incurable pain.

Arthur Frank, in *The Renewal of Generosity,* speaks of generosity as the hallmark of a fine physician, residing in "the grace to welcome those who suffer."[23] That is exactly what my fine doctors do. They are glad to see me. Their faces light up. Every minute of our appointment is a fully attentive one that makes the visit seem much longer. The last time I saw Dr. Ko before I moved to Victoria, he drew a sad face at the end of my file, which he showed me with a soft smile. It warmed me no end. It told me what Dr. Yasin's warm smile and handshake tell me. These are physicians who look for a sense of community in their work. They are not just "providers" of "services."

In every culture there are rituals of touching to show that the other is welcome. A young doctor I tried out for a possible family doctor when I first arrived in Victoria, stepped into the examining room, my file in his hands and said, "What's the matter?" He didn't so much as shake my hand or look me in the eye. I felt insulted. There was no going back to him. When Dr. Yasin shakes my hand, with his welcoming smile, at every appointment, I relax. When Dr. Ko let his hand rest on my shoulder or arm between injections, I felt a healing energy. When he gently put his hand on my shoulder when I broke down badly one day in his office, I felt a deep sense of comfort. When you have been in chronic pain for years, you feel you have become "untouchable," as Dr. David Kuhl puts it. He adds that "through touch—both touching and being touched—a healing process begins.... Being touched and being in touch are experiences of the present, experiences of now."[24] True touch grounds you. Life returns. It makes you into a normal person. Genuine physical touch counteracts aloneness in a deep sense that cannot be accomplished by words.

Dr. Lewis Thomas, the former president of Memorial Sloan-Kettering Cancer Center in New York, wrote that touching is a real professional secret, an essential skill, and "the most effective act of doctors."[25] After almost two hundred and fifty visits with twenty-two doctors and specialists in eleven years, I would not have known that if it hadn't been for the exceptional Dr. Ko and Dr. Yasin. But doctors can't touch a person with sensitivity if they consider the patient as only an object for their diagnostic gaze. The two do not go together.

Patients bear the burden, says Dr. Kuhl, of a doctor's own unresolved psychological and emotional issues about death, pain, suffering, and relationship.[26] Then he adds:

> If as a physician I have not asked myself questions like: *What would my life be like if I were told today that I had a terminal illness? Or…What would I feel if I knew that the usual course of the disease I just learned I had is rapid and includes considerable pain or discomfort?* then I might talk without empathy or sensitivity.

Dr. Michael Stein asks similarly, "How can a doctor understand the terror, loss, or loneliness of a patient if he can't imagine it for himself?"[27]

My family doctor wants me on morphine again. I panic. He knows that a year earlier I had been prescribed morphine and the side effects were horrible.

"For the rest of my life?" I ask, holding my breath.

"Probably," he says, his eyes on my file.

Just "probably." Nothing else. I sit there, silenced. Oh God, please, no. I can't have my brain fogged over for the next thirty some years. But I said nothing, because he said nothing. His eyes did not meet mine. I sensed him steeling himself, shutting himself off. Dr. Kuhl may be right: this doctor may not have dared to ask himself the question what it would be like for him to suffer from constant pain, losing his job, his social life, having to go on morphine.

Dr. Steven Aung, recounting his conversation with the Dalai Lama, notes that in the Buddhist tradition, physicians provide a blessing along with their treatment—a normal and essential component of primary care.[28] The blessing conveys "loving kindness" and implies the wish for peace and recovery. The doctor-patient relationship entails "good friendship" between them—that is, making patients feel at ease, inspiring respect and trust, providing appropriate counsel, being a good and tolerant listener, and explaining things clearly.

One day, the tragic situation in the Middle East came up in my conversation with Dr. Yasin, a Muslim, born in Libya. "It must be hard for you to follow what is happening there," I said.

"Yes. I pray a lot," he replied, then added pensively, "but I also pray for my patients. Every time I put a needle into you, I pray I will do it right." His words stopped me in my tracks. A blessing with every needle. A doctor praying that he may do me no harm. The active spiritual aspect, if present, rather than an essential aspect, is a personal commitment in Western science where, as Cassell phrases it, "the promise...is that the knowledge does the work."[29] But it should be an essential aspect.

Patients can be devastated or braced by a turn of phrase, says Jan Hoffman in the *New York Times*.[30] It took me a long time to believe my prolotherapist and wellness physician when they told me there was a chance for improvement. Every time I thought I was getting a bit better I would think, "Wait, I can't be getting better, for X, the important pain specialist said we were running out of options. And Y, the neurological specialist said I would be in serious pain for the rest of my life. And surgeon Z said my life was ruined. How can I be getting better?"

Hoffman notes how difficult the language of hope has become. But he says a consensus is building on at least two fronts: that what fundamentally matters is that a doctor tells the truth with kindness and that a doctor should never just say, "I have nothing more to offer you." Palliative care physician David Kuhl, referring to those who are dying, tells his fellow physicians never to say, "There is nothing more that can be done for you."[31] I was told that by several physicians and specialists while I still had some thirty years to live. The worst error a physician can make, says Dr. Atul Gawande in *Better: A Surgeon's Notes on Performance*, is "giving up on someone we could have helped."[32] In the domain of chronic pain, I feel quite certain that error is made far, far too often.

Medical students learn about broad ethical principals. But do they learn what Arthur Frank refers to as "microethical" decision making, which he sees as a continuous flow of "moral moments?"[33] Did the resident pick up on the fact that it was not smart on the part of the surgeon to talk to me about my "ruined life?" Did he think of what happened to me as a result of what the surgeon said or what he did to my neck? Or had he already learned to "minimize thinking" so as to "conserve energy," as one doctor cited by Frank said he was told to do in medical school? I would not be surprised if my not-so-good doctors thought they were having a good relationship with me. When the knowledge of science is seen"to do the work," the fact that they were adding to my suffering, I suspect, passed by them.

In contrast, when Dr. Ko would quietly say, "I know…" when tears filled my eyes as I tried to speak of my pain, and how he would not try to minimize my suffering in any way, I felt an immediate relaxation come over me. Whereas the words, and behavior, of my not-so-fine doctors sent the message that their science was right, yet my body was a failure in its lack of response. Dr. Ko's "I know…" acknowledged my altered life in pain as well as the limitations of his science.

Thankfully, as the March 29, 2006 PBS program *The New Medicine* showed, some medical schools have started to add communication-and-listening skills to their curriculum. By 2011 all new medical residents will have to exhibit empathy while examining an actor posing as a patient. In a pilot program at Harvard Medical School students are paired with patients and trail them through their medical procedures and interactions with doctors to counter what Dr. Barbara Ogur, in an interview with Nathan Thornburgh of *Time,* calls "ethical erosion," referring to the desensitization to patients' suffering as a result of the pace and pressures of residency.[34] And as a medical student in this program says, this isn't "squishy science…it's a way to get the kind of results everyone wants from the medical system." However, as another physician tells Thornburgh, it will take more than curriculum reform to get patients the care they deserve. If doctors only get a minute and a half with a patient, this physician says, then whatever they learn about patients' needs isn't going to matter a lot. Lack of empathy on the part of doctors is also tied to systemic problems.

What do you do as a person in chronic pain when your doctor or specialist has nothing to offer you, doesn't listen, or has made your pain worse, either by intervention, by doing nothing, or by his or her behavior?

It is the middle of August 2001, and I have an appointment at the pain clinic of the medical school at a university in the Netherlands. With the help of my daughters, I had returned to Holland to say good-bye to a dying relative. A week into the visit I suffer a severe pain attack. Through connections at the university, I am given an appointment with the director of the clinic. He seems eager to tell me what they do. I had hoped to learn something new, but all he has to offer is the TENS machine and the drug Rivotril, which he says, they find very successful with patients with pain problems such as mine. Using TENS involves applying electronic pads to the painful areas and regulating the strength of the electronic pulses as needed. I was given the unit to take home for a two-week period. Two weeks should tell.

Then the director spoke with some irritation about patients who engage in what he refers to as "doctor hopping." That is "*niet goed,*" he says. No good. You need to stay with the doctor you have and persist with the treatment. I used the TENS machine twice daily for two weeks. It felt pleasant enough but did nothing for my pain.

Had I stayed with my first family doctor and the neurological specialist he sent me to, I would have had only temporary relief from severe pain by relying on pain medication, massage, and acupuncture. Had I stayed with my anesthesiologist, I would have had annual repeats of the nerve-burning procedure, risking developing nerve pain, or alternatively, been on daily morphine. Had I stayed with what another doctor and another neurologist advised, I would have been on morphine, possibly for the rest of my life, and no one would be trying to figure out what else to do.

The American Pain Foundation's pamphlets *Finding Help for Your Pain* and *Reading This Could Help Ease Your Pain* contain strategies for interviewing doctors and becoming your own advocate. Chronic pain sufferers are urged to educate themselves, to be persistent, and, if necessary, to change doctors. The pamphlets note that many doctors still see pain as a side effect of other diseases and may not recognize chronic pain as an illness in and of itself. If your doctor can't help you, is impatient, doesn't believe you, doesn't listen, or only knows how to prescribe drugs, it's time to move on.

To keep searching for professionals who can bring about relief is hard work. It often seems like too much. Many a time, I haven't wanted to see anyone, ever, anymore. And for weeks I don't. But somehow, I keep my ears open: I hear about a new specialist in town. A new pain clinic. An excellent meditation class. Dr. Ko's words always are somewhere in my head: "Lous—never give up!" And that includes doctor-hopping when needed.

5 Pain Medicine

On Opioids, Pain "Killers," and "Side" Effects

I would not have survived without opioids. I am grateful that my medicine cabinet contains opioids in the prescription drugs Tylenol 3 and Percocet, and that during the worst of years I had Dilaudid and morphine to fall back on. A twenty-two-year-old Victoria woman suffering from severe chronic pain told me her doctor refuses to prescribe opioids for fear of making her addicted. I almost wanted to give her mine. According to many pain specialists, addiction to opioids when prescribed for pain is, in fact, very infrequent.

It is unbelievable to me that doctors are arrested by the U.S. Drug Enforcement Administration (DEA) for prescribing opioids for pain in ways the organization does not agree with. The Pain Relief Network reported an increase in the suicide rate among chronic pain patients following the DEA crackdown that has been going on since early 2000.[1] I would have been one of them had doctors not prescribed opioids for me. Not relieving pain, says David Morris, "brushes dangerously close to the act of willfully inflicting it."[2] To me, it *is* willfully inflicting it.

A 2005 policy analysis by the CATO Institute in Washington, DC, says the DEA's painkiller campaign has cast a chill on the doctor-patient candor necessary for successful treatment.[3] Of course. It has also scared many doctors out of the field of pain management and likely persuaded others not to enter it, thus, the report concludes, worsening the already widespread problems of undertreating pain.

My own problem has been not the danger of addiction but that the adverse effects of opioids are too serious for constant use. Nor do they completely eliminate pain, as Fishman also notes.[4] As Mary Carmichael reported in *Newsweek* on June 4, 2007, almost 200 million prescriptions for opioids for pain relief are written in the United States each year, but fewer than a third of people on opioids report any relief. They do not work well for all of us, but they are absolutely necessary for many. For state policies to interfere with the medical use of opioids is to invite desperate acts by those in pain and shows complete ignorance about the living hell that is chronic pain. In a consensus statement, the American Academy of Pain Medicine, the American Pain Society, and the American Society of Addiction Medicine conclude that state policies should continue to address issues of prescribing opioids that may contribute to drug abuse and diversion but that they must not interfere with the medical use of opioids.[5]

With regard to what is involved in prescribing pain medication in general, the learning curve has been steep for me, and my experience has been very problematic for a number of reasons. From my interactions with other pain patients, I find my story to be typical. Five related aspects stand out: (1) the still widespread assumption that painkillers are the only or at least the best way to manage pain; (2) the trial-and-error approach to prescribing painkillers; (3) what patients are told and not told about these medications; (4) painkillers rarely kill; (5) and the meaning of "side" effects.

If one has a conventional doctor, as I did at the time of the accident, he or she will put you on some common pain medication. That will be essentially it. Many doctors were taught to see pain as a symptom of an illness or injury to be suppressed with drugs. "The biggest single problem," Dr. Ellen Thompson, pain specialist at the Ottawa Hospital, told Holly Lake of the *Ottawa Sun* on October 16, 2005, "is that pain [as a pathology itself] is not something that is taught in medical school." Noting there were more lessons about malaria than pain she said, "I'm still waiting to see my first case of malaria." "There is no correlation between what's taught in medical school and the prevalence of a complaint," said another physician. Dr. Mailis-Gagnon, in that same interview, claimed that most health-care professionals do not understand how the mind-body-emotion connections play out in chronic pain and, therefore, will never understand pain.

Those doctors who do understand pain will prescribe pain medication, but they will also discuss alternative approaches to pain management. This would include a referral to a comprehensive pain clinic—if you are fortunate and there is one where you live—where medical/surgical interventional approaches are available but also alternatives such as acupuncture, prolotherapy, gentle chiropractic work, neural therapy, dry needling into trigger points, and biofeedback. They may even have someone who specializes in teaching stress reduction or mindfulness meditation; a psychotherapist who specializes in pain; and someone who knows how nutrients affect the way neurotransmitters, hormones, and other chemical processes interact with the body's pain pathways.

"I didn't know that there were pain doctors or anything about pain medication," says Mary Vargas, a lawyer suffering from chronic pain.[6] I am a university professor. Neither of us had any knowledge of pain specialists and pain clinics, and we knew nothing about pain medication. Knowing about these things is a matter of experience, not necessarily of level of education. I think doctors tend to forget that.

I had no idea prescribing pain medication is entirely a matter of trial and error. Or how many different kinds there are. "Now I have more than fifty medications to pick from," says pain specialist Russell Portenoy.[7] "I have no way of knowing which a patient will respond to, so my approach is one of trial and error." I had naively assumed there were specific medications for different kinds of pain and that doctors knew what they were doing. Mine acted that way. Initially, I'd leave the doctor's office, prescription in hand, with a sense of relief. Now I would be free of pain! It wasn't until I read Dr. Fishman's book *War on Pain* that I learned the true nature of the beast. Arriving at the right drug, he says, is a "tricky business."[8] One of the doctors interviewed by Marni Jackson told her it could take a year of "tinkering" with different combinations and doses of drugs to find the right one.[9] Most doctors, he added, do not know this. If they don't get immediate results, they bail out. I am now in my eleventh year and still do not have the "right" drug. But the questions for me are: What is the "right" drug? How much pain should I tolerate? How many adverse effects should I tolerate?

My psychotherapist had a helpful response to the question of how much medication I should take. His answer: "It depends what kind of experience you want to have." Refocusing the question on the kind of experience I want to have on any given day allows me to focus more on the present and on the purpose of my day. When the pain is intense, I have no choice. On days the pain is less severe, and I have time to be very quiet, to meditate, do the body scan, massage my painful neck, and do gentle stretches, I can discharge pain without medication and live with what I cannot discharge while feeling good about not poisoning my body that day. I have been told by pain physicians that I need to take medication systematically, not only as needed. There should always be medication in your system. That makes sense, of course, if medication is seen as the only way to pain relief and alternative approaches are not considered. I am not against medications per se, and still take plenty of them, but the short- and long-term adverse effects pose serious problems that I want to avoid as much as possible.

Over the span of eleven years I have been on the anti-inflammatories Toradol, Celebrex, Vioxx, Arthrotec, Feldene, and Voltaren; the painkillers containing opioids Tylenol 3, Percocet, M-Eslon, Dilaudid, and Tridural; the muscle relaxants Flexeril and Baclofen; Imitrex; Risperdal (a drug developed, not for pain, but for schizophrenia and bipolar disorders); Inderal (a beta blocker developed for hypertension); the antianxiety and muscle-relaxing drug Valium; the anticonvulsant drugs Neurontin and Topamax, as well as Rivotril (developed also for panic attacks); and Imovane as a sleeping aid. Because some antidepressants share nerve pathways with pain, I was also put on the antidepressants Elavil, Norpramin, and Celexa, all having severe adverse effects. Now, as I write, I take, depending on my circumstances, Tylenol 3, Toradol, an occasional Percocet, Imovane, Valium, and Baclofen, as well as plenty of over-the-counter ultrastrength Tylenol. I stopped taking the others due to their severe adverse effects or because they did nothing to relieve my pain. None of this is to say that some of these drugs may not be working well for others. I am illustrating the trial-and-error nature of prescribing painkillers, the fact that many do not help, and the many adverse effects they can cause.

Initially, when drugs only dulled the pain, if they worked at all, I was surprised. Weren't they supposed to kill it? When I told my doctor, he said, "Yes, there will always be some pain. The pain does not entirely go away." "You feel pain slide from unbearable to bearable." says Dr. Fishman.[10] When in severe pain, that's about it. And "bearable" does not mean you can ignore it.

The serious adverse effects of my taking properly prescribed pain medications include the following: severe drowsiness, agitation, rebound headaches, considerable stomach pain, nausea, vomiting, serious constipation, increased depression, heightened anxiety, and cognitive disturbances (in my case, the inability to put words to thought, confusion, impaired short-term memory, and hallucinations). Strangely enough, some of these adverse effects were the very thing the drug was supposed to stop. I mentioned that to my pharmacist. "Yes," he said, "that's the way drugs are. Every drug has the potential to make the very thing it is [supposed] to correct worse."

Morphine was the worst. It caused extreme constipation. Overwhelmed by pain, I had not noticed I had not moved my bowels for several days, which created a huge and painful problem. If only my doctor had warned me…I could have easily taken a strong laxative along with the morphine. According to Fishman, the one predictable side effect in all patients on opioids is constipation.[11] And, he says, it never goes away. Constipation is such a consistent outcome that if a patient is not constipated, Fishman wonders if the dose is sufficient. Every one of his patients on opioids is also on a laxative. Of the three doctors who prescribed daily morphine for me, only one mentioned in passing the possibility of constipation, but even he said nothing about what to do about it. I was left with the impression it would be no more than a minor problem.

Worse than the constipation, morphine brought on violent hallucinations at night. During the day, my mind was a dense fog. I moved in slow motion. There was a pervasive sense of being absent. I couldn't hold a thought. I started to substitute words, saying "Zuzuki" instead of "jacuzzi," "root" instead of "food." I started a sentence and couldn't finish it, but started another sentence instead. At first my daughters laughed, but it quickly became clear it was no laughing matter. I stayed with the morphine for almost three weeks. It didn't get any better. I told my pain specialist. He denied it could be that bad. He told me that he had two hundred patients on morphine and they were all "doing fine."

Part of me sympathizes. This doctor was trained in a certain way. He saw as his task to suppress his patients' pain. Nothing he had tried worked. *He* was running out of options. But how did he know for sure that his two hundred patients were all "doing fine" on morphine? Were they telling him the truth? Or was he dismissing their complaints just as he dismissed mine, as he did not know what else to do? Had he ever been on morphine himself? Pain is what the patient says it is, and adverse effects are what the patient says they are.

I told my psychotherapist, a former nurse in a terminal cancer ward, that my specialist did not believe morphine caused my hallucinations. "Oh, yes, they do," she said, and took out her medical encyclopedia. "Here it is…hallucinations." A fellow chronic pain patient told me he had lowered his morphine dose and was trying to get off it altogether, as he thought he was going crazy. Alphonse Daudet described his experience:

> Effect of morphine.
> Wake up in the night, with nothing beyond a mere sense of existing. But the place, the time, and any personal sense of self, are completely lost.
> Not a single idea.
> Sense of EXTRAORDINARY moral blindness.[12]

My experience exactly. And Daudet was on morphine for a long time. He never got used to it. A number of those that Rosenfeld interviewed spoke of long-term fogginess, the slowness of thought and speech that comes with morphine and other opioids.[13] It's like having a mind of "fogged glass," one of Michael Stein's patients told him.[14] Thoughts come in slow motion—thought and language, no longer clearly connected.

These are not side effects. These are effects that alter life in major ways. As Kabat-Zinn notes, a principal source of disorder and disease *is* disconnection, meaning the inability to attend to relevant feedback from the body.[15] As *Newsweek* also reports, many pain patients on morphine stop taking it because, as with me, the adverse effects interfere with living.[16] So, the question for me always is, Do I want my mind distorted and have less pain, or do I try to put up with the pain so my mind stays clear? When the pain is severe, of course, my mind cannot stay clear either. Then I may as well take opioids. None of this is to say that opioids may not be the best solution for a number of people to dull the pain. I recently met a pain patient for whom morphine is working just fine; his pain is dulled, his mind is clear. But opioids are not necessarily the best route for everyone.

Often it is not until doctors themselves become ill that they discover what their patients experience. In a moving account, psychiatrist Dr. Nanette Gartrell tells how she started taking the antidepressant bupropion for panic attacks and suffered from severe side effects that increased the very symptoms the drug was supposed to correct.[17] Ever since then, she describes potential side effects to her patients in much greater detail and switches medications immediately when they occur. "In the past, I would have encouraged the patient to stick it out....I wonder where I'd be now if I had followed my own advice."

A psychiatrist I saw to help me sort out my medications diagnosed severe depression and suggested I try an antidepressant. I told him that years ago I had been on Serzone for seasonal affective disorder, and it brought on terrifying sudden suicidal ideations. After the accident I had been put on desipramine, which kept me wide awake for forty-eight hours straight. This kind man then put me on Elavil, which was far too sedating. Then he put me on Celexa, which made me vomit violently over a period of twelve hours. I phoned him. Had I taken it with food he asked. No. It did not say so on the bottle. He had not said so. The pharmacist's printout did not say so. He apologized that he had not told me. He then said, "I would like you to go to a drugstore and buy Zantac to settle your stomach. And then I want you to be brave and continue with it." Right then I experienced another wave of nausea and said, "Sorry, I have to throw up again" and hung up on him just in time to get to the bathroom. I decided I did not have what it took to be brave.

The struggle with adverse effects is exhausting. I don't think most doctors have any idea what it means to deliberately risk—by swallowing that little pill—inflicting even more misery of one kind or another on a body and mind already in pain for years. Or perhaps they do know—but don't know what else to do.

To take side effects seriously would bring down pharmaceutical companies' profits. It has been a shock to learn about, what Stephen Hall (in a review of books by Marcia Angell and Jerry Avorn, respectively the former editor in chief of *The New England Journal of Medicine* and a professor at Harvard Medical School) refers to as the "stomach turning" details involved in the "systematic obfuscation of risks" too many companies engage in, and of the huge numbers of illnesses and deaths occurring from properly prescribed drugs.[18] The volume of bad news—mind boggling to anyone—is particularly nerve-racking for those of us taking these drugs. And taking drugs is a *huge* part of the daily lives of chronic pain patients. When my doctor now wants to try out a different pain medication, I get nervous. How can I trust my doctor's knowledge when it comes to drugs? I can't. And that is not because I don't trust my doctor.

Doctors' off-label prescription of drugs is particularly scary to me. I used Neurontin and Topamax, developed as anticonvulsants; Inderal, developed for hypertension; Risperdal, developed for schizophrenia and bipolar disorders; and recently I walked out of a pain specialist's office with a prescription for Mirapex, a drug developed for Parkinson's disease. It was the first prescription I decided not to have filled. After ten years of unsuccessful experimentation to find the "right" drug, often experiencing adverse effects that add exhaustingly to the pain I already have, and reading about the many possible risks of severe long-term effects, something inside of me said, "Enough!" It is enough. A guinea pig no longer.

And then there is Tylenol. Recently, I came across a series of warnings that made my heart sink.[19] Figures of how many people end up in the emergency room from acute acetaminophen poisoning vary from 15,000 to 55,000 a year. Over three hundred products contain acetaminophen, and most people—that included me at the time—have no idea how much acetaminophen the products they use contain. In terms of Tylenol's dose-related risks, I don't drink alcohol or fast, conditions that increase the danger of acute poisoning. But during the worst years, I often swallowed, day after day, more than the recommended dose, which is easy to do when hellish pain refuses to go away. Regarding long-term effect, I have reason to worry after eleven years—and highly likely many more to come—of almost daily use of Tylenol. While 4,000 mg is the daily maximum dose noted on the bottle, the *American Journal of Respiratory and Critical Care Medicine* has linked long-term daily or frequent use of as little as 1,000 mg acetaminophen (just two extrastrength tablets) to respiratory illnesses such as asthma, chronic obstructive pulmonary disease, and decreased lung function. Other studies note high blood pressure and kidney damage as long-term adverse effects. What, then, is safe to take—for the long, long run—when a person is suffering from chronic pain?

I assume doctors are meant to warn you of the possible adverse effects. But do they? I was not told Serzone could bring about suicidal thinking. I was not told Celexa could make me vomit violently for twelve hours. I was not told that desipramine could leave me wide awake for forty-eight hours. I was not told morphine could bring on severe constipation, hallucinations, and severe language-thought disturbances. The shock of experiencing these *effects* added to the pain I was already experiencing. In all these years, only my present family doctor, a complimentary physician, has expressed concern about drugs' adverse effects. He is the first doctor who periodically orders a blood test to check the health of my liver.

Easing Pain without Medication

Often the adverse effects of drugs are preferable to the pain. But as both short- and long-term adverse effects started to present a real risk to me, and the best that drugs can do is to temporarily dull the pain, I began to look for alternatives.

The Wellness and Hormonal Connection

In summer 2002 I was so exhausted and run down that my body would walk itself to the couch several times a day. Yet, not one of my doctors had pointed out the connections among certain nutrients, hormonal levels, and pain. It wasn't until I saw my wellness physician that I found one who did. But when he suggested bio-identical hormones, I resisted at first, and it took some prodding on his part to get me interested.

"But you might feel better," he said. I thought he was nuts.

"How can I feel better when there is all this pain? Just take my pain away—then I will feel better!" He more-or-less ignored my comment and ordered a blood test to measure the major hormones estrogen, testosterone, progesterone, DHEA, and thyroid. All were way below the average levels for my age. I had hardly any left. Small wonder my energy sources were depleted.

He also suggested protein supplementation. When his advice indeed resulted in much more energy and endurance, I was happy and told him so. He just smiled. I am very grateful to him for putting up with me.

This doctor did not focus narrowly on my pain, trying to "kill it" or "conquer" it with drugs or other chemicals. Instead, he focused on aspects of health that influence pain and its consequences through alternative routes, suggesting a gentle weblike metaphor in which many aspects of health intersect with the chronic pain experience. It now all seems so obvious. Yet no other doctor or pain specialist addressed these matters. I had to find a wellness physician, and pay his fees myself, to get important help that any of the other doctors could have easily provided, for none of it is very complicated.

The Mindfulness Meditation Connection

Mindfulness meditation is the actual practice of being rooted in the present. Being mindful calms the mind and emotions. It softens the pain and gives it a different quality. When a person is in chronic pain the nervous system is fired up, and meditation provides a dimmer switch to turn the firing down. Meditation is now a daily practice on my part, almost a way of living, softening pain as tensions of body, mind, and emotions rise less quickly and stay more often below the pain threshold. Although mindfulness meditation is grounded in Buddhist tradition, one doesn't have to know anything about Buddhism to benefit from the practice. Kabat-Zinn's books and CDs, with their down-to-earth approach to mindfulness, have been very helpful for me.

A related form of meditation involves what I think of as my "disappearing act." This is difficult to describe. I am on my back and my attention (not my thoughts or feelings) is on my body. Doing this lets go of past and future. There is nothing in my mind but the feel of my body. I let my attention go from feet to legs, hips, chest, neck, shoulder. Momentarily I become this body, as it is all that lives in my attention. Then, on the out breath I do nothing when my out breath comes to its end. I do not breath in. Nor do I hold my breath. There simply is a "gap," a space where nothing happens. My chest feels as if it has caved in just for a second or two, bringing about a feeling of depth, deep inside. My mind is no longer active. It has dissolved into a peaceful nothingness. I control nothing. I am not there. "I" have disappeared.

Then, out of nowhere, my legs will shake. My shoulders. My arms. Often all at the same time. Sometimes gently. Sometimes almost violently. It is like an electrical discharge that I can actually *feel*. A current leaves my body. A deep release of tension. If I am in pain when I do this, the pain softens. It took a long time, bit by bit, to learn to let go of the contents of my mind to allow the body to discharge itself in this manner. For as long as the mind is busy, it will hold the body in tension, supporting pain. With chronic pain, one's thoughts, emotions, and fears are all woven tightly into the chronic pain experience. Mindfulness and attentiveness practices empty all that, even if only for seconds or minutes at a time, bringing down tensions, softening pain.

Then the "gap," that peaceful space, passes and my chest, on its own account, breathes in again.

The Naturopathic and Homeopathic Connection

A naturopath diagnosed a stressed liver, stressed adrenal glands, and a sluggish lymph system—all courtesy of years of pain, drugs, and stress. I took several naturopathic products for three months to correct the problems and started taking even greater care of what I eat and drink. That means food and drinks that increase the health of the immune system and the natural pain-fighting systems in the body. I also take several nutritional supplements—glucosamine, MSM (methylsulfonylmethane), omega-3 fatty acids (the good fats that help lubricate my joints and nourish my brain), and a high-quality multiple vitamin and mineral supplement. These supplements repair critical tissues and some have natural anti-inflammatory properties. The American Pain Foundation website also identifies a number of nutritional means to counter pain.

The National Institutes of Health (NIH), through its National Center for Complementary and Alternative Medicine, divides complementary or alternative medicine into five broad categories: (1) Mind-body healing that focuses on using the power of the mind to improve health (meditation, prayer, music therapy, visualization); (2) Alternative medical systems that have developed apart from the mainstream biomedical approach (acupuncture, homeopathy, and naturopathy); (3) Biologically based therapies that use natural substances in healing (herbal products and food supplements); (4) Body-based or manipulative practices that promote healing by moving one or more parts of the body (chiropractic, massage, and osteopathy); and (5) energy therapies that tap the body's energy fields (the hands-on healing practices of Reiki, therapeutic touch, and magnets).[20]

I have used almost all of these approaches, and collectively they have increased my endurance, softened the pain, and shortened recovery time from pain attacks. They help to keep my emotions and my mind in check. None have had any adverse effects, either short or long term. Taken together, these therapies impact both the generation and continuation of pain and how people experience and manage it. Unfortunately, prolotherapy—which has been of significant benefit to me—is not yet mentioned by the NIH.

I did learn that there are often different schools within each alternative approach. For instance, the first two chiropractors I saw cracked my neck and back. The chiropractor who works with my prolotherapist adjusts my atlas bone using gentle pressure only. Of the two osteopaths I saw, one practiced more like a chiropractor, cracking my back, the other gently manipulated my skull in a way I found similar to the treatments of the craniosacral therapist. It is important to try out different practitioners within the same profession, asking questions, comparing them to each other, and somehow deciding who can help best based on one's sense of what the body can absorb without harm, what brings relief, and the therapist's skillfulness at what he or she does.

There are now various multimillion-dollar research projects focused on mind-body research funded both by the U.S. government and private foundations. At least one leading managed-care organization (HIP USA) has started to cover some mind-body practices, as does Medicare if they are administered by psychologists.[21] Mind-body medicine is seen by Dr. Herbert Benson as "a saner starting place" for treating illnesses made worse by stress, as chronic pain surely is. He says, "If it fulfills half its promise, it could reduce medical cost while improving our health and our lives. And whatever its limitations, it has the advantage of doing no harm."[22] Such treatments are also important because, as Dr. Buckenmaier points out, the body has many ways to get information about pain to the brain—a safety mechanism in itself. If the brain doesn't hear from one modality about injury, it will hear it from another.[23] To stop pain, says Dr. Buckenmaier, we must get at it at different levels with a variety of methods that act through separate mechanisms. Simply using pain medication only attacks the pain via one channel, which is not enough.

It wasn't until recently that I *felt* how the body channels pain through several different pathways. Through mindfulness meditation, I have come to observe how my thoughts, attention, and emotions can increase or decrease pain. For many years I thought that there had to be one method out there, somewhere, that could get rid of my pain entirely. But all paths (physical, emotional, mental, chemical, psychological, social, and spiritual) must be walked. The Arthritis Foundation sees the doctor of the future as knowledgeable about both alternative and conventional medicine. I now have a family doctor and a pain specialist who use both approaches. I feel at ease with these doctors. All options are on the table. I know I am in good hands.

6 *On Science and Time*

Science: The Question of Parameters

A mutual friend asked me to talk to a young woman, a mother of two young children, who had a serious accident resulting in neck injuries similar to mine. She cannot hold up her head—something I remember all too well—and is in severe pain almost constantly. I urged her to see my prolotherapist to stabilize her neck. Although my prolotherapist is an experienced pain specialist, her family doctor refused to write the needed referral because, she said, there were no double-blind studies on prolotherapy. (There are.[1] There are also many publications of clinical studies.) "Let's wait," the doctor told the young woman. Wait for what? For things to get worse and worse, and for the pain to become its own pathology? I begged her to change family doctors.

"I can't do that! I have been with her for years. She delivered my children!"

"But she's not going to do anything for you other than prescribe drugs—she has no clue what else to do, right?"

"True, she said that herself."

"Who is ultimately responsible for your well being? For getting rid of your horrible pain?"

The question takes her by surprise. There is a long silence. "*You* are," I say. "Not your doctor. Your doctor does not want to look any further than what her training has taught her. You are responsible for what happens next."

Once again, I beg her to change family doctors. She will not hear of it. Plainly, this is misguided loyalty to her doctor and indirectly to science. But it is one, I fear, engendered by the authority the scientific method bestows, which reflects the experimental view of how pain can be subdued. But there are other equally important ways to understand how pain can be eased. When doctors are trapped in science, and science has not yet addressed certain therapeutic possibilities, there is a chance their patients are trapped in pain. "To seek certainty itself," says Eric Cassell, "is ultimately to abandon the patient."[2] I have felt abandoned in this way many times.

As a patient, I find it ironic that doctors adhere to the scientific method for exclusive guidance even when there can be no actual certainty. There is, indeed, only a *seeking* of certainty but not a capturing of it. After all, the scientific method deals with hypotheses and probabilities. Not with life in all its complex manifestations. To limit treatment of chronic pain exclusively to these parameters can be detrimental.

One of my specialists openly acknowledged the uncertain nature of his work. You have to imagine, he explained, that our work is like a multilevel highway interchange, roads circling around each other, above and below each other. We can only guess: maybe the problem is there, or here, or over there. We may be right, we may be wrong. But that is all we can do. Given that only weeks earlier he had put large needles into my neck at five different places to burn my nerves (which temporarily made the pain worse and also gave me horrible nerve pain for six weeks), I walked out of his office in a daze.

Dr. Mailis-Gagnon has this to say:

> We misdiagnose, under-diagnose, maltreat and undertreat pain. We plague patients with unnecessary narcotics when there are better alternatives or we deny medications when they are needed. We try to determine underlying physical disease...but ignore illness behavior, and on the other hand, we miss significant organic causes and send the patient to a psychiatrist or psychologist.[3]

Marni Jackson, who attended the 1999 World Congress on the Study of Pain, noted how some surgeons admitted their own failure, particularly in the treatment of back pain.[4] "Surgery is not the answer for back pain, and it doesn't work," one well-known surgeon said. At the congress, alternative treatments were completely absent or only marginally represented. Yet alternative approaches, as Jackson also states, are for a good many of us our lifeline, often bringing more relief than drugs and surgery.

Jackson further notes how completely out of the picture the real patient was at the congress. She points to the irony that the scientific study of pain has created communities of researchers and physicians who discuss their papers in an upbeat manner, their presentations infused with humor, while those in actual pain suffer from increasing isolation. We are typically isolated as well from these conferences. But we should be there. Literally. We can bring with us the reality of how our lives have been altered by pain and how we find relief from both pain and suffering in ways that lie both inside and outside of conventional science. As people living in pain, we need to be educated by the knowledge rendered by science. But scientists and physicians need to be educated by knowledge rendered by our lives—knowledge that is different, but of equal importance.

Also, we cannot forget that even medicine's scientific approach is muddled with political and bureaucratic mingling. For instance, David Leonhardt points out that under the current system, no one is paid to come up with the right diagnosis.[5] Medical professionals are paid to perform tests, do surgery, and dispense drugs. There is no bonus for a cure and no penalty for failure, he says, except when the mistakes rise to the level of malpractice. Though Leonhardt's observation was obvious once I read it, it was a revelation to me. It may in part explain the many contradictory diagnoses I received, some of them made with confidence, others made almost in a guessing manner. None of my doctors was paid to come up with the right diagnosis or the right treatment. Instead, they were paid just for treating me, even when their treatments were based on an incorrect diagnosis, did not help, or made my pain worse. I think most patients are not aware of this state of affairs that reflects the "standard of care" rule. That is, as long as a doctor is using the same therapies other doctors are using, then mediocre results are acceptable because everyone else is getting those same results. This allows for inappropriate treatments to continue. The casualties of all this in the domain of chronic pain are all around us.

In my case, had I received a *wide* range of treatments directly following the accident, I am certain my chances for recovery would have been much better. As Thernstrom observes, every chronic pain patient is a testament to the dangers of the conservative wait-it-out approach to pain.[6] The body's pain system is plastic and therefore can be molded by pain to cause more pain. With prolonged injury, progressively deeper levels of pain cells in the spinal cord are activated. Ongoing pain, Fishman similarly states, can have a profound effect on the brain architecture.[7] An acute injury sets off a barrage of pain signals, which causes nerve cells in the spinal cord to sprout new connections, which in turn intensify the pain signals. By intercepting the barrage of pain signals at an early stage chronic pain might be prevented. Unfortunately for me, my family doctor at the time of the accident took the "let's just wait and see" approach. And, of course, back then, I myself knew nothing about the complexities of chronic pain.

Regarding surgery, in the residential pain clinic I attended I met one young woman who had twenty-three back operations and was still in severe pain. Another person had six operations with equally negative outcome. Melanie Thernstrom reports on how often surgery leads to new or worse pain, an outcome for which, patients told her, they had no warning. David Morris notes that between ten and twenty operations for the same problem is not uncommon, and that certain operations leave patients worse off.[8] The American Pain Foundation similarly cites many stories by chronic pain sufferers having undergone many surgeries resulting in no improvement or, in some cases, in increased pain. I heard one of my pain specialists tell a colleague that he had just seen a new patient who had had thirteen operations on her neck (several by the same surgeon who wanted to cut into my neck) and who was still suffering from severe neck pain and headaches. Dr. Fishman refers to the "failed back syndrome" as an "all too common condition of persistent or worse pain after surgery and other treatments that were supposed to help."[9] The phrase "failed back syndrome" in itself is curious to me, as it suggests the failure of the operation can be put on the patient's back, as if it always belongs there. A more appropriate phrase would be "the failed operation syndrome." What does it mean for surgeons to be accountable? More of the same treatment that hasn't worked is not an effective or even a rational way to proceed.

With regard to nerve-burning procedures, Fishman notes how more often than not the severed nerve grows back, making new connections, and may even transmit more intense pain than before.[10] My case too. In the field of neurology, burning and cutting nerves is done in the belief that the problem lies in the peripheral system and that nerve impulses from the site of damage, the periphery, transmit pain to the brain. To stop the pain, the signals coming from the periphery must be interrupted. Hence nerves are cut or burned by neurosurgeons, or blocked by anesthesiologists with chemical compounds. Both were done to me. The pain should stop, but it often does not. Pain symptoms simply change locations, or the pain can get worse.

The more recent view, known as the centralist model, assumes that once the pain has become chronic, the central nervous system has started to generate pain on its own. Chronic pain, then, is the disease itself, no longer a symptom. The problem, as Fishman points out, is that now the brain that must make sense of the pain is the same brain that generates it.[11] Damaged nerve fibers and a damaged and altered nervous system create their own experience.

For some of us, both the peripheral model and the central model may be playing themselves out simultaneously, but it is the dominance of the peripheral model that is called into question.

None of this is to deny that some pain patients are helped by mainstream interventions. And if a intervention becomes available from within conventional parameters that looks promising for me, I might go for it, but only after deliberate research into adverse effects, success rate—and the chances it could make my condition worse. Given the many failures and the risks these interventions pose, however, alternatives should be tried first. This is not a naive patient attack on science. Without science medicine would collapse. But there are ways of knowing that cannot be captured by the scientific method. People living with chronic pain suffer and can be abandoned in those cases where their pain cannot be helped within the parameters of conventional medicine and nothing else is offered.

Time: The Medical Slaying of Minutes

A chronic pain patient tells me her doctor brings her timer with her and sets it for eight minutes: the end of the appointment. My pharmacist tells me that his doctor has a sign on his door that says: "Only one question per visit." In February 2008 I needed to consult a new doctor. A sign in her waiting room said: "Please, only one complaint per visit." Complaint. I thought: Is that how this doctor will see me—as someone who complains?

And if I were to ask her for medication for my pain, am I then not allowed to mention a stomach ache that has been bothering me? Particularly with complex chronic illnesses, how does a patient delineate "one" question or "one" complaint?

Shortly after I moved to Victoria, I had my second appointment with my new family doctor, and I had a lot of questions. The first appointment had been short: mainly to communicate the basics. For this one, I am scheduled for a long appointment to discuss my many problems. We are doing just fine, when, as I ask a further question, he says, "No, no more. Another question would financially jeopardize me."

What did he say? I am taken aback. Up to this point he seemed pleasant enough. Now I'm not sure. Perhaps it was all a performance.

"But I thought this is a long appointment."

"It is, but time is up."

There was no warning that we were almost out of time. I did not know how long a "long appointment" was. I was learning what this man had to offer me. I left his office upset. How dare he be so abrupt and so blatantly financially motivated? How demoralizing for both patient and doctor to be counting seconds and dollars.

I knew I had to tell him how I felt, otherwise I would no longer be comfortable seeing him. At my next appointment I told him I had been taken aback by his bringing up his financial concerns. He blushed and ran his hand through his hair.

"But time was up."

"But I didn't know that. You were *very* abrupt. So how many minutes do I have with you?" His answer is vague. His posture is defensive.

"But how many minutes?" I insist. After all, how will I know when to stop if I don't know how long an appointment is supposed to be?

"Ten minutes."

"OK," I respond. Deeply frustrated with the conversation, I decide to let it go at that.

It is possible that his comment about his finances was some kind of humorous attempt to get me out of the door, because he turned out to be a much nicer fellow than forecasted by that encounter. If so, it is a sad testimony to the fact that doctors, having to count minutes, feel they have to engage in such tactics.

The need for dialogue when it comes to chronic pain, as contrasted to acute pain, is urgent: pain patterns can change, the effects of drugs can change, other difficulties in life compound the severity of the pain, alternatives need to be explored. The nerve center that produces the chronic pain experience is in effect a network, linking components—language, memory, emotions—from virtually every region of the brain. What was "just" pain has taken over an entire life. Treating chronic pain as an acute matter—the "here are more drugs" kind of appointment—is totally inadequate, even damaging.

The moral demand of dialogue, says Arthur Frank, is that each party grant equal authority to the other's voice.[12] Having to set one's mental clock for only a few short minutes makes dialogue nearly impossible. Dr. Radomsky recounts her extensive and empathetic interactions with her pain patients.[13] She couldn't possibly have limited her interactions with her patients to eight minutes, which is often noted as the average time a doctor spends with a patient. Dr. Peter Salgo, a professor at the Columbia University College of Physicians and Surgeons, notes seven minutes as the average time mandated by U.S. publicly traded HMOs.[14] Doctors feel powerless to change things, says Salgo. He then argues for a "patient driven" revolution that would change this slaying of minutes. I took his words personally. My reaction was one of amazement: even while living in constant pain, not only do I have to learn as much as possible about my condition so I can sort out the unbelievable amount of conflicting information I receive from doctors, but I now *also* have to bring about a revolution in the system so doctors can spend more time with me!

The tension between minutes available and the more extensive time needed for understanding the complexity of chronic pain also shows in the 2006 American Pain Foundation's publication *Treatment Options: A Guide for People Living with Pain*. On page 4, the APF states: "The impact of pain requires an understanding that the whole person experiences pain: that is, the mind, body and spirit." On page 5 the patient is urged to write down all questions he or she has, because, "you may not have much time with your provider."

Constrained to just a few minutes, the "whole person" is the first casualty to fall by the wayside. For myself, with the majority of my doctors, the pervasive time pressure has been nerve-racking. I prioritize my questions at home. I reprioritize them in the waiting room. I prioritize them again in response to what the doctor says, quickly deciding which questions to pursue and which to drop. This is hard to do in any situation, but when in pain it is impossible, and I invariably leave feeling defeated, forced to act content with much less than I need to know for my own comfort and understanding. And while I realize that a full explanation may not be necessary, the answers I receive to my questions typically barely scratch the surface.

"Listen to your doctor," admonishes the pharmaceutical poster on the back of my doctor's office door. But an equally important consideration for those who chronically live with pain is "Does your doctor listen to you?"

Some observers have called for primary-care doctors to be paid by the hour. As it is, a doctor gets paid the same whether the patient is a basically healthy person with a bit of the flu or a person with a serious chronic illness. In the United States experiments are under way to increase pay for family physicians who devote more time and attention to their patients—in order to save the system money, as it is assumed extra time will improve the quality of health care.[15] In these experiments physicians are also getting paid more for caring for someone with a chronic illness and for caring for patients by phone and e-mail.

"Time is money" has been carried to a destructive level. In any rethinking of pain management, time—its nature, its value, and its meaning—must be a central focus. That, and the long-term cost of rushed, piecemeal appointments, in terms of dollars, but—speaking from personal experience—also in terms of increased suffering.

7 *Pain and Others*

My Taxi Driver

It was fall 1999 and I had to fly back to Toronto from Seattle where I had visited my daughters for a family emergency. On the flight out I had gone into a major pain attack, which is a horrible thing to experience. Buckled into a narrow seat there is nothing you can do but take one pill after another. So I was very nervous about flying back. Fortunately, I experienced only mild pain, kept under control with Tylenol. At the airport I took a cab for the drive home. Sitting in the back seat of a cab has its own problems. Backseats slope back, which makes it difficult to keep my neck straight. I have to lean forward to speak to the driver: head forward, chin forward—a killer for my neck. So I drew directions on a piece of paper and handed it to the driver before I got in. He was in his mid-thirties, spoke with a heavy accent, and appeared exhausted. The collar of his coat was wrapped high around his neck. I told him why I had drawn directions for him.

It turned out that four years earlier he too had had a car accident. Cold weather made his pain worse, he said, just as it did for me. He took Toradol, which gave him stomach pains. He had a young family to support and had to keep working. I asked him about his doctor. "He gives me Toradol," he said, "and then tells me, 'Come back next month.'" He had had no physiotherapy, no massage, no acupuncture, nothing. I asked if he had seen a specialist? "A specialist?" he asked. "Why?" He did not know there were pain specialists or pain clinics. Was the car insurance paying for anything? No, he had signed off under pressure not knowing what else to do. Did he have extended health-care coverage? No. I sat on the very edge of the backseat, holding on to the seats in front of me, trying to keep my back straight. Here we both were. So similar in pain. So different in how we were treated.

I urged him to ask his doctor to refer him to a pain clinic. I told him of the pain clinic I went to. I wrote down names, phone numbers, the address. I did all this with a sense of foreboding. I had no trust his doctor would be willing to refer this man to a good clinic. Since he had not done so in four years, I felt confident he had no plans to do so any time soon.

When I think of my taxi driver I feel a sense of unearned privilege. As an assertive Caucasian professional woman, I was sent to the best specialists my doctors could think of. I have good extended health insurance. He is an immigrant, his English not that easy to understand, totally dependent on his family doctor who is doing nothing for him.

Richard Payne, chief of Pain and Palliative Care Service at the Sloan-Kettering Memorial Cancer Center in New York, summarized the data on the role race and ethnicity play in the management of almost every clinical setting, including the management of pain.[1] At least nine studies document racial and ethnically based disparities in access to pain medications and outcomes of pain treatment. He concludes that "patient profiling" must be raised as a major problem. In a position statement, the American Pain Society likewise concludes that racial and ethnic minorities are at risk for problematic access, poor assessment, and inferior treatment.[2] Given that unattended pain can quickly become chronic, this puts minorities at additional risk. "You can't get into the heads of individual physicians to see what they're thinking," says Gary Puckrein, president of the National Minority Health Month Foundation, "but, on the whole, it's clear they're not managing pain as aggressively in minority populations."[3]

No kidding. I met my taxi driver before I read these studies, but I knew right away that our race and socioeconomic status directly led to a difference in attention, treatments, and referrals we received from our respective doctors. Apart from systemic racism, says Payne, cultural and linguistic differences (which includes inadequate knowledge about the medical system) and whether people are assertive in asking for needed referrals and treatments are also a factor. Dr. Mailis-Gagnon adds to this her overview of research findings that show the impact of the ethnic identification of the physician on assessment of pain and mode of treatment.[4]

Diane Hoffmann and Anita Tarzian summarize research with regard to gender documenting that women are more likely than men to be under-treated or inappropriately diagnosed for their pain.[5] Women are more likely to be given sedatives for pain while men are more likely to receive pain medication, suggesting that female patients are more often perceived as anxious rather than in pain. Also, attractive female patients were thought to be experiencing less pain than unattractive ones. The researchers concluded that the association of beauty with health influenced health-care providers in assessing pain.

I can relate to this from the patient's side: when I have a medical appointment on a good day when I look more rested, I worry more that the doctor won't believe me. Even my choice of clothing is a conscious decision—if I have the desire to dress well, the doctor might decide, however unconsciously, I can't be in that bad a shape, not understanding that my desire to dress well can be an expression of exactly the opposite—being in bad shape and desperately wanting to feel better. Dressing nicely to feel better may be a particularly strong need in women compared to men. Given that most physicians and pain specialists are men, they may not be conscious of such desires and therefore may misinterpret the meaning of a woman's appearance. Race, gender, appearance, class, ethnicity—all can influence health-care workers' perceptions in assessing and treating pain. There is much work to be done in raising awareness in these matters.

"What do you do all day?"

The assumption by others about all this free time I have since I am not working is a stark indication of the lack of knowledge that surrounds chronic pain. "Are you going to travel?" "Are you going to teach at the University of Victoria?" "How about visiting us—we'll pick you up in Atlanta, and the drive home is only about five hours."

It is November 2002, six years after the accident and before prolotherapy brought partial relief. For months on end, I have slept for no more than four of five hours a night. The devil wakes me up. The days are shattered by unpredictable pain attacks that last for hours. Exhaustion rules.

"What do you do all day?" a former colleague who phoned me asks.

"I have pain. I manage pain. I see doctors."

"Oh," she says after a moment of silence, "but what do you *do* all day?" Now that I was no longer working, her mind could not fill in the gap with the word *pain,* and with the fact that serious ongoing pain erases your day. Before the accident I, too, would have wondered what a person with chronic pain would be doing all day.

"What do you do all day?" an acquaintance asks. She looks puzzled.

"I struggle with pain. I see doctors and therapists of one kind or another. I try to do the basics in the house. I have to move around carefully so as not to throw out my neck. That takes about all the time and energy there is."

"Oh…" she says. She tries to understand, but looks puzzled.

In Victoria, I attend a dinner with colleagues from the university. A light headache and a sore neck are under control with Tylenol 3. The wife of a colleague I had met years ago says, "My husband told me you don't work anymore since your accident. I have been wondering—what do you do all day?"

I don't know how to explain my life to people who ask me what I do all day. I had no idea what "pain management" was before it took over my life. The whole day at home. How boring. Pain meant something you put up with till it passes. Everything else stays the same. With chronic pain, nothing stays the same. But others have no way to understand that. The problem with chronic pain, says David Morris, is that its presence is undramatic.[6] It does not grasp the imagination. It is so treacherous, he says, because it works almost totally in secret. There is no visible deformity. No outward sign of damage:

> Chronic pain patients tend to move in an in-between realm: they clearly are not well, but their malady will not let us see them as absolutely sick. An affliction that operates in-between and in secret, of course, generates endless paradoxes. How can we combat an epidemic so clandestine that no one (except its victims) really notices it?

A chronic pain patient, who can no longer work because of her pain, told me she was asked the "What do you do all day?" question at her car insurance hearing. The question—seemingly so straightforward—stunned her. She couldn't answer it. Finally she said, "I may go for a walk" and immediately knew her answer might be held against her. The problem is that the question as asked *assumes,* unproblematically, that you have "all day" to be active, to do things. The phrasing of the question is generated from within the context of the questioner's life. It implies that someone who is not working because of chronic pain has all day to do things—just like anyone else. The question needs to be something like "Can you describe what your day is like?" or "Can you describe how your pain limits your days?" Such questioning would acknowledge the altered nature of our lives.

What do I do all day? Not much. Yet a lot. The next time someone asks what I do all day, I will refer them to these pages. A pained life poured into a book. Why I cannot come along on a day trip. Why I cannot teach. Why I cannot fly from Victoria to Atlanta and take a five-hour car trip. Why I have to cancel a dinner date. These questions are also a stabbing reminder of what I used to do, and still long to do. I have given up expecting others to understand. Only those few who have been with me for several days at a time come to understand the limitations of my life. The woman who shared the house I rented in Victoria when I first arrived told me after a few months almost in disbelief, "I have not seen you one minute without pain." That is what I do all day.

Friends: In how many ways do I now know them?

I used to feel fortunate to have a number of very good friends in my life. But I never could have imagined how friendships would be put to the test by the disaster that befell me. How my concept of friendship would have to change. It has been among the more difficult consequences of living with chronic pain.

I have experienced the loyalty of a few, the falling by the wayside of several, including some I considered close friends, and the fear of making new friends because once they know of my pain, they too may fall by the wayside. The books on chronic pain I've read, and testimonies by chronic pain patients I know, describe the experience of losing friends and the resulting descent into loneliness:

> The friends that were there are no longer there. The family that was there is no longer there. The long relationship is no longer there. I'm a different person, totally different.
>
> Catherine Berardenucci, CBC *Ideas,* "The Culture of Pain"

Lous, the phone never rings anymore.

> thirty-two-year-old woman with severe chronic pain

Chronic pain is an insidious disease that can infiltrate your entire life....Every day I meet people whose feelings of hopelessness, rejection, anger, and anxiety rule their lives.

> Scott Fishman, *The War on Pain*

Will I ever have a boyfriend again?

> young woman with chronic pain

Friends hang in there with me as best as they can, but that is not very much.

> forty-year-old man with chronic pain

Pain is always new to the sufferer, but loses its originality for those around him. Everyone will get used to it except me.

> Alphonse Daudet, *In the Land of Pain*

They just don't understand.

> woman with chronic pain

Friends drop like flies.

> APF website, "Voices of People in Pain," Joey's story

Our stories of lost friendships are heartbreaking. As we receive fewer visits and phone calls, the despair over a lonely present and an equally lonely future hovers darkly. Friendship becomes complicated. For me, when in pain, a visitor has to be a good friend with whom conversation flows easily, because the effort to engage in small talk with more superficial contacts often increases pain. But cutting out casual contacts also increases isolation. As there are unspoken rules for social interaction, and those in chronic pain can no longer meet them, the descent into loneliness becomes unavoidable.

To this day I still don't know how much I can tell others about this pained life. I follow my instinct of the day. The most important ingredient in any friendship for me has always been a high degree of honesty. At first, my words about my troubles came out as a stream, unstoppable. Initially, friends, family, and even some colleagues were all ears. But soon, it seemed, most had heard enough. They may have felt helpless. I may have bored them. I could even hear myself becoming boring, not to myself, but to them. They needed to talk about something else. For me there wasn't something else. Pain had erased the something else. Pain had become the always present and always urgent center of my attention. They would talk about their lives with the flutter of words that once were also my words: their jobs, their social lives, their travels. I wanted to grasp a friend's arm and hold on, so I would be pulled in her direction, into her activities, her enthusiasms, which once were mine too. But I felt myself sinking further and further behind, stuck in a place of which they knew nothing. Yet that place was now my life.

A director of advocacy in a pain clinic says society refuses to face the horrors of chronic pain, saying, "Don't look over that edge. Look over there instead, at something cheerful."[7] And yet, she says, what those in pain want is someone who will stand next to them and say, "God, that looks pretty scary."

Marni Jackson carves out the poignant truth about the effect of chronic pain on others: "It leaves a stain on everyone who lives with or comes into regular contact with someone who copes with chronic pain."[8] A stain. The metaphor shocks me because I know it to be so. After listening to someone who lived with severe pain, Jackson wrote, "I began to experience what many people feel when confronted with the inconsolable: I wanted to leave." Reading her words, I am all the more conscious of my predicament when I am with others. I do not want to be a stain. But it is part of the disease.

Over time something else began to grow in me: the wish not to be a burden. The wish not to add to the stresses in another's life. How to reconcile the two needs, one for attentive friendship, the other not to be a burden? I feel my way through it from moment to moment, probably erring on both sides at different times.

Only the very few "eccentric" ones, as Hermione Lee puts it, understand that I can no longer fulfill my part of our friendship as I used to.[9] They have kept in touch and have carried the burden of friendship. Those friends I will cherish forever, as I will some new friends who have become friends knowing of my pain. Paradoxically, when with these friends, there is less of a need to talk about my pained life. I know they will listen when I really need them to.

I now try to accept the fact that when friends cannot handle the life I now must live, it does not mean they were not good friends within the former context of our lives. I try to accept that when my car crashed, all my relationships profoundly changed—relations with my children, with a partner, with friends, with colleagues—and future relationships, relationships I fear because I can no longer sense what may or may not be possible with someone new. Sadly, all this comes at a time when the need for human contact and support is intense.

I now understand how it is chronically ill people develop inferiority complexes: "No one wants to be with me. I am no longer good enough." In my desperate moments I think this too. This is one of my journal entries before prolotherapy brought back a measure of social life: "I tear up at the strangest moments. It comes from such loneliness and despair. With this pain, will I ever be able to enter into anything with anyone? People will stay away from me. Who wants to be friends with someone who is in constant pain?"

In *The Nature of Suffering*, Eric Cassell makes the point that social life and the rules for social participation normally override the inner needs of the individual.[10] While the acutely ill are often relieved of these rules, he says (as I understand it, this is so because everyone understands acute pain and it is assumed to be temporary), the chronically ill rarely are. However, says Cassell, the chronically ill are not able to sustain the behaviors that the rules for social participation demand except at great cost. Following these rules requires focus and energy that those in chronic pain no longer have. Indeed, my social life dissolved altogether during the worst four years, for exactly the reasons Cassell mentions. Even now, when I force myself to participate in social life while in pain, I cannot meet the social requirements for participation for any length of time without ending up in greater pain. The conflict between the demands of social interaction and the needs of the chronically ill and pained person is heightened, notes Cassell, even to the point they threaten to tear the person apart, and as a result the chronically ill must learn to live with themselves. During those worst four years, that was my life—living with myself, except for occasional company of the few good friends who did not give up on me altogether and visits from my daughters who, though living hundreds of miles away, came as often as they could. I wrote in my journal: "Finally, I am resigned to being alone.... The starting point now, each day, is to be alone with this pain."

Looking back on those worst years, I panic. I freeze. It must have all happened to someone else—it couldn't have been me.

Paid Friends

During the worst years of daily pain, the names of people written on my calendar were nearly exclusively those of doctors, specialists, and therapists of one kind or another. Month after month. As friendships fell away, some of these professionals provided the sense of community I had lost.

The minutes I spent with my favorite pain specialist in Toronto, the sympathetic Dr. Ko, provided a much-needed human connection. So do my visits with my favorite masseuse in Victoria, Lynn Smith, with whom I engage in easy talk during the massage. Dr. Nasif Yasin, my prolotherapist, is another compassionate doctor who never seems rushed and who takes the time for friendly exchanges. I trust these professionals realize that their time with those isolated by chronic pain serves a relational function.

One very important person in this regard is my psychotherapist, Brian Grady. He is the most vigilant listener I have ever known. Once I moved to Victoria, I knew I had to find someone to unload on. I needed to hear myself talk. Inside my own head I was going around in maddening circles. I tried out six therapists before I found Dr. Grady. It turned out that when it comes to chronic pain, psychotherapy rarely speaks directly to relentless pain and its consequences.

I found Dr. Grady in the Yellow Pages. As I was looking through ads by therapists, I found his was the only one that had the word "pain" in it. I wasted no time making an appointment. He was younger than I expected. I felt a twinge of disappointment. Once more, I thought, this is not going to work. I could be his mother. He won't be able to handle me. But within minutes, I knew I had entered a different therapeutic environment. I felt safe and at ease. It turned out he is a Buddhist and practices meditation. If there is one word to describe my experience of this therapist it would be *present*. This was more than sympathy or empathy. It was vigilance, attentiveness, and being completely rooted in the present. Present with me for the entire hour.

I never feel that some particular theory or approach is more important to him than I am. Nevertheless, he has a PhD in clinical psychology and ten-years experience working in a pain clinic. He is also an acupressurist—that is, he doesn't use needles—and knows Chinese medicine. Yet, he doesn't force his views onto what I tell him.

He listens. Occasionally he will mirror and summarize what he has heard me say, and he hears everything I say. From time to time he interjects a thought, an observation, a practical suggestion. Never a judgment. At times he even senses what I am trying to say but am not able to articulate. It is miraculously freeing to be with a professional who really wants to understand—my devastating experience is worthy of being understood. There is no need to protect myself, hold back, or watch out for comments that inadvertently trivialize my pain. He does not pretend to understand when he doesn't. He continues to listen instead with a puzzled look in his eyes that encourages me to try harder to explain.

When I admire his ability to fully listen, he reminds me that he is taking his cues from me, because at my first appointment I had told him I came because I needed to hear myself talk and needed someone to listen. Taking his cues from me! In my experience with therapy, this is unusual. When trying out other therapists I felt that my words were habitually transposed into the theories they believed in. But I did not want to be theorized. Before any theories could ever make sense to me, I needed someone to whom I could bring the torment of my life as I knew it and who was able to listen to it in a sustained way.

Dr. Grady leaves me my truth: he does not change it for his own comfort. He does not steel himself against my suffering, as I feel too many of my health-care professionals have done. On the contrary, I sense he engages his mindfulness practice, before I knock on his door, to be aware and open to the moment whatever it might bring. I can use my words as a direct translation of my thoughts and emotions. I am safe. I can be truthful. This also means everything comes out. The deepest despair I can put words to. His attentiveness allows me to think better, to find words that speak accurately. My tears flow. Not needing to stop them, he gives them his full attention as well.

I trust him. I ask him questions born of fear: Am I crazy? Am I exaggerating? Is my life not as difficult as I say it is? I tell him how I feel more isolated when people say "But you are handling it so well" or "But you look good." I tell him that at times I think I am mentally unstable. Maybe I am going crazy.

His response is immediate. No, you are not crazy. You are perfectly sane. You have gone and are going through immense difficulties, and anyone would suffer as you do. You are not exaggerating. Your pain is exhausting as it would be for anyone. It would be unbearable for anyone. He looks at me directly while saying all this. He is passionate. He means it. He understands.

My relief is immediate. I believe him. I leave his office feeling a weight has been lifted from my shoulders. Someone understands me. Here is this person, this stranger, in whose presence I am what I am. For many others I am a "stain" as Marni Jackson put it—I can only be with them if I hide the pain. Dr. Grady is someone for whom I am *not* a stain. For a full hour I am a whole person. "You are welcome here," he said a few times, "with all that you bring with you, with all of your pain." My emotional reaction to these words is sharp and swift. I choke up.

I tell him a major question now is, what is my task in life? He has no specific answer. Yet, his being so attentive to all I say and making the saying so easy allows our sessions to clear my head and ground my emotions. I know that only I can figure out where my life can still go. What his attentive listening does, however, is to let me hear my own deepest thoughts, fears, and longings, which in turn adjusts my perception of the parameters of my present life. This process helps me respond to my own questions. And that is much.

One day as I get up to leave, I tell him I don't know how he does it: listening so completely, without judgment or interpretation. He takes in my words. A brief pause. Then he says that for him to be a witness is also a part of his own education as a human being. Our sessions educate him. I felt deeply moved. For a therapist to be a witness is what those living with serious pain need more than almost anything else.

But he is also one who may disappear. Who will be gone if the money runs out. Who will be gone if I move. If he moves. Not a real friend. Yet, somehow, more than a friend.

My task is not to confuse what these fine professionals do with friendship, although the mind at times wants to go there. This is made easier by my knowing that the therapeutic effects of these "paid friends" will last long after the therapy is over. As someone said, when a person truly listens, you will carry her or him in your heart for the rest of your life.

Suicide: "Let's not go there."

We are running out of options.

pain specialist, 2001

…a ruined life…

neurosurgeon, 2001

She will never be able to return to her previous teaching position.

report, family doctor, 2001

Her problems are of a permanent incurable nature.

report, family doctor, 2001

We need to go to morphine.

pain specialist, 2001

The prognosis is poor. Ms. Heshusius has a condition which has no definite treatment and tends to slowly worsen over time.

report, pain specialist, 2001

…a disability of a permanent incurable nature.

report, family doctor, 2002

There is no cure for her problems.

report, family doctor, 2002

These problems tend to get worse.

report, pain specialist, 2002

You need to be on long-acting morphine.

family doctor, 2002

I agree with putting her on morphine. There is no cure.

report, neurological specialist, 2002

No more options. A ruined life. It is 2002. I am still in Toronto. I have had many drugs, nerve blocks, Botox injections, and my nerves are burned. Nothing helped. Open neck surgery is too risky. I am put on morphine. The only means for real pain control left is to end the life of this mangled neck altogether.

"Let's not go there," the masseur says, as he briefly lets up massaging my shoulders and back that feel like steel. His words are immediate. I haven't quite finished my sentence. We speak easily during the massage. I often will say aloud whatever thoughts go through my mind. A man my own age, totally professional while totally compassionate. As his hands tell my muscles to let go of spasms, his mind continues to be responsive to anything I say.

Except for this moment. It is the end of a desperate week of intense and constant pain. A bit fogged by painkillers and frantic from exhaustion, I say, "I am at the point where I really want to die. Just to take a few bottles, lie down…"

"Let's not go there," is his immediate response. His voice is definite. *He* does not want to go *there*. But I do. *Someone* needs to know my deep, ongoing thoughts about ending my life, the freedom from pain and despair it will bring, and what stands in the way. This exhausted soul of mine speaks hesitantly now; sensing if I can get him to "go there" with me. Please…listen. He changes the subject.

Chronic pain is so "ruthless," so "relentless"—words Scott Fishman's patients use—and so psychologically devastating that sufferers will try anything, Fishman says, even risking total paralysis or death.[11] The desire for death can become like a "primitive drive" as, indeed, it became for me. There comes the moment that the need to end the relentless pain is absolute. The need becomes so intense that the connection between ending pain and dying as a result is no longer in one's awareness. When pain stabs you front, back, and center, day after day, month after month, and no one can stop it, you yourself must stop it. *Stop it.* What happens after that is not your problem.

I told five other health-care professionals of my suicidal despair, hoping that receiving some compassion and understanding would enable me to gain some strength, some reason to want to stay alive. These were their responses:

Number one: Completely ignored my words.

Number two: I broke down when I said the pain had been so bad I no longer wanted to live. He glanced up, bent over his file again, wrote something down, but said nothing. When months later I saw a copy of his report he had sent to another physician, he had written down that "she wanted to do herself in."

Number three: Said nothing. When I received copies of his notes later on for insurance purposes, he too had written that I had mentioned I wanted to end my life.

Number four: Never said a word. The questionnaire I had had to fill out before the first consultation with him asked this question: "If it were in your power, how many years do you still want to live?" I was nervous. I was not sure if I could trust this new doctor enough to talk about it. I was convinced he would pick up on my answer that during the long stretches of constant pain I no longer wanted to live. He greeted me perfunctorily, picked up the questionnaire, glanced at it, and asked, "Is there anything else you want to tell me?" I was stunned.

"No, didn't you read what I wrote?"

"Yes," he said. No more. Not a hint of concern. When I learned later this doctor gathers data for research purposes, I had to consider that my nervous admission on paper may have served as just another entry into some data base. I felt betrayed. I felt treated like a child that had said something not worth responding to. There was no validation of any sort, though he himself had asked the question.

Number five: Merely nodded his head and said, "I'm putting you on Prozac." Drugs, drugs, drugs. I heard the same subtext: Let's not go there. Let's chemically cheer you up instead.

Only recently, my new masseuse and my family doctor in Victoria picked up on my dwelling on death, although I didn't express these thoughts nearly as strongly as back then when I was still in the throes of despair. However, I deeply appreciated their sensitivity and courage to show their worries, and I wished my doctors back then had done so when suicide was constantly on my mind.

As psychotherapist Miriam Greenspan observes, to admit that unhappiness might be justified would undermine the entire rationale of the medicating mind-set.[12] When the psychiatrist ordered me to take Prozac and I refused, he was not pleased. I asked him if he wouldn't feel despair were he in my shoes. He looked surprised, and then just shrugged his shoulders. I guess I was not allowed to be depressed about a matter that is worthy of depression. Greenspan echoes exactly my own view: "I'm not opposed to the wise use of antidepressants, but doing so in a medical model, in the absence of any validation for the emotion itself, can make despair's journey seem like an absurd exercise in anguish to no end." The refusal of my doctors to validate the torment of my life by not responding to my expression of suicidal thoughts pushed me deeper into the very anguish I was seeking to release. "First, do no harm," also refers to what is not done, to what is not said.

The truth may have another side as well. Quite possibly, all took my words seriously, but none had the courage to respond. For in the words of Dr. David Kuhl, it takes personal strength and courage to stay with a patient's dark emotions:

> I am afraid that if I get too close, then I might have to experience aspects of *his* life that are very sad, unjust, complicated, and unfixable. I'll be helpless in the face of tragedy, far too aware of the limitations of the science of medicine and my personal inability to cure, fix, or repair his suffering and death. I'll feel like a failure. I'll experience grief—an emotion I would rather avoid. Besides, there is no place or time in my schedule for processing emotions.[13]

But *someone* should have been willing to go there with me. One would expect at the very least a referral to a good specialist in posttraumatic stress. I didn't get any. I had to find one myself. Shouldn't physicians have a list of names ready for suicidal patients? "Medicine," says David Morris, "seems instinctively to flee from tragedy....Overwork and pragmatism cannot fully explain the tendency of medicine to pull away from the subject of suffering."[14]

I also approached a very close friend; he, too, did not want to "go there." One person, only one, went there with me—one of my daughters. She even courageously initiated the conversation. A hidden wound finally was exposed. The reasonableness of my suicidal preoccupations was acknowledged. She listened. She witnessed. She did not steer me away from my dark thoughts. At least not initially. I broke down. Sobbing in her arms, I slowly moved into a blank space where the darkest emotions were washed away for a moment, having been allowed some of their redemptive stirrings to surface. I heard myself say, "I am so afraid....I am so afraid." I finally could speak the fear that had tormented me—the fear that I would have to go on living this way indefinitely.

But then, she also wanted me to go on living: "What about me? You would not see me anymore! I love you mam! You would not see your kittens anymore." I realized that even she could not fully understand how peaceful the thought of death had become. How desirable. How imperative. How could I explain to her that my death wishes bore not on my love for her but on the unbearableness of constant pain and the prospect of much more of it for years to come? How does one explain a terror that is not explainable in language and that is not known in the other's experience?

Then she said words I will take deep down with me into my grave: "I'd give you all the money I have in a heartbeat if it would make your pain go away. I want you to live. I would give my arms if it would make your pain go away. If someone could cut off my arms to make you better, I would do it." She paused a moment, and then she said, "But not my legs. I have thought a lot about it, but I couldn't do without my legs." With tears flooding her eyes she added, "I have to be able to walk, but you can have my arms." Her face had turned white. She was so earnest it cut through my soul. I do not know if I myself could be that big. The sobs that come to the fore when I write this down again, three years later, I do not quite understand.

Of the medical books on chronic pain I have consulted, only Dr. Fishman's gives suicide serious attention.[15] References to suicide are even absent from self-help books in which negative thoughts about one's situation are typically seen as problems in need of a positive makeover. Even in the ten-day residential pain clinic, to be happier seemed the goal of all activities and group counseling, and the staff's own stories about their personal experiences with chronic pain were all, without exception, uplifting restitution stories. As suicidologist, Toyo Fuse, states, "the biggest hurdle for the suicidal is the taboo-nature of truly discussing the problem openly and honestly."[16] Even my doctors conspired to maintain this taboo. One would think the fact that the suicide rate for those in chronic pain is two to three times higher than for the average population would be enough to take suicidal wishes expressed by a chronic pain patient seriously and to be open to talking about it.

Chronic pain is not terminal, though it can be permanent, unbearable, and is *always* near. A kind of death. As Dr. Albert Schweitzer said, pain can be worse than death. Suicide presents itself as a liberator. For me, the worst of hell passed about two years later as the strengthening of my ligaments began to stabilize my neck, softening the pain. Thoughts of suicide eased. But mine is a narrative I could easily not have been around to tell.

Regaining Community

Eric Cassell speaks of the great isolation and loneliness inflicted by severe illness and chronic pain: "The first step [to restore health] ... is to reach out to the suffering person to bring him or her back with the rest of us."[17] Social contacts, he says, "must be facilitated." While at first his words sound so right, Cassell does not tell us how that might be accomplished, and why others would invite us back while the very problem that got us excluded in the first place has not changed. What would have to happen to be invited back into social life while still in pain?

In my experience, and from what I hear from other people living in pain, part of the problem is that others invite you to join in *their* activities (and stop inviting you after you have had to decline a number of times). But for the most part, we cannot engage in their activities. In my case, I cannot go on a day trip or long hike or any hike if it is not on even ground. I cannot go to a movie in a regular theater (the psychedelic and obnoxiously loud previews throw my brain into panic and into pain); I cannot go for the whole day to Vancouver to visit a museum, have dinner, and go to a concert; I cannot go on a weekend trip filled with activities. I cannot just go to any restaurant—anything too busy or with pop music is out. It is a rare person who makes the connection that what is needed is to invite someone in chronic pain to do something that can be done within the limits the pain poses on their world.

Instead of the regular movie theater, many cities have at least one specialized theater that does not play previews. A day trip may mean one activity only, going through the day as slowly as needed. A dinner party at someone's house needs to be a relatively small and quiet gathering, and so forth. I think that many people would be quite willing, at least once in a while, to adjust their social life to meet these limits if they would only think of doing so.

However, it is also true, as Virginia Woolf observed, that true sympathy is hard to come by, burdened as people are already with their own sorrow.[18] Sympathy, she says, is "uneasily shuffled off for another time." The comfort she found herself came from the sky, from clouds, from flowers: "It is in their indifference that they are comforting."

It is with those things of beauty that are indifferent to my life that I find my day-to-day sense of belonging. I don't make them uncomfortable with my pain. They don't leave because of my pain. They bypass the conflicting human needs and emotions. My cats are that way. Their absolute otherness safeguards the integrity of the self I was, am, and will be: they do not mistake one for the other. Unlike humans, they do not enter my world of pain and compare the self they find to the self they knew or want to find. People often confront me with the fact that my pain creates social spaces that are nearly unbridgeable. My cats simply meet the self I am at any given moment. My behaviors when in great pain or in great despair have become a normal part of the household scenery for them. As Dr. Michael Stein said of his brother who was dying of cancer: "Only his cats could be counted on."[19] The irony, of course, is that my cats do not make me need humans less. The fact that on a day-to-day basis they are now my major source of companionship and affection, reminds me starkly of the human isolation the pain has wrought.

How does one make friends when chronically living in pain? I struggle with the answer. I meet someone new. We agree to meet for a coffee. I hear Marni Jackson's words in my mind: You are a stain. I think: Be pleasant. Don't talk about your pain. Just mention in passing—you may have to cancel at the last minute, at times you have pain—I'm sure I will make it, but just in case—oh, from a car accident—yes, it was terrible but it's getting better now. I hate my instinct to pretend to be better than I am when meeting someone new.

Pretending is never necessary when in the company of other people who live with chronic pain. In the summer of 2006 I joined a pain support group at the Royal Jubilee Hospital Pain Clinic here in Victoria. This interdisciplinary clinic is the most patient-oriented pain clinic I have attended—by that I mean that patients at this clinic are treated as equals with the staff, as intelligent adults who know a great deal about their pain condition. Many group activities are offered that are organized around patient-to-patient interaction, and although the waiting time to see a doctor is at least a year, patients can start the group activities right away. I have attended a series of educational sessions and am now attending a weekly meditation class. There is a sense of freedom when you are with others who understand your life, with people who nod their heads when you speak about your pained days. And when others speak, it feels like coming home. I belong some-where. Here, I know who I am. Here, I can relax. Here, it is peaceful.

Yet, the desire to be part of the larger community remains. The improve-ment resulting from the prolotherapy made it possible to slowly begin to regain some sense of community, although I rarely make commitments for both the afternoon and evening on the same day. I would pay a price for overdoing it with a major pain attack. Regaining community under these conditions is difficult and takes time. There are now some friends in my life. People who have become friends knowing that I suffer from pain. I will forever think gratefully of them.

8 Where Are We with Chronic Pain? A Patient's Perspective

Chronic pain has recently been on the radar of the media. For instance, *Newsweek* (May 19, 2003; June 4, 2007), *Time* (February 28, 2005), and NBC's *The Today Show* (March 28, 2005) have featured special reports. Newspapers such as the *New York Times, USA Today,* and the *Ottawa Sun* all have reported on chronic pain, often more than once. I am glad to see that chronic pain is finally on a map that is accessible to everyone. But there remain some concerns.

First, the emphasis is almost always on trying to get rid of pain. But for many of us the pain cannot be made to go away. Second, with some exceptions, media reports are often sprinkled with unrealistic claims and hopes. Pharmaceuticals under development are often spoken of as if they might be the next miracle drug: we have heard this now so many times. Those who are mentioned as having their pain taken away miraculously by surgery are the exceptions. These surgeries wouldn't work for everyone even if everyone had access to them, which they do not. Third, access to good pain-management programs mentioned in these articles is poor and differs greatly across populations and demographic areas. And further, the emphasis is too often on how the biomedical model views and treats pain. While the importance of alternatives has started to be acknowledged, in most instances, I believe, it has not been stressed nearly enough.

The Scientist, in a March 28, 2005, special issue on chronic pain, offered a tempered assessment based on the views of a number of well-known pain specialists. They conclude that those studying pain are getting a better understanding of what causes pain but that they cannot necessarily fix it. They emphasize that the adverse effects of drugs are a "tremendous barrier" to effective treatment. Nor are drugs by themselves sufficient. Says one specialist: "There are a multitude of specialized receptors in skin and other tissues that signal chemical, thermal, and mechanical changes associated with pain. We know…that targeting only one of them will not work…blocking the actions of any one of them will likely lead to compensatory effects in others."[1] Several of the authors conclude that we need to study the less well-known aspects of chronic pain—the social, cultural, and personal dimensions that interact with pain mechanisms. Exactly.

Claudia Wallis, writing for *Time,* concludes that there are many ways to temporarily relieve chronic pain and increase the quality of life and that drugs and surgery are not necessarily the best way.[2] Nor the most economical. Though drugs will always be an important part of pain management, the quest for pharmaceutical salvation seems, so far, to be misguided. Roughly half of chronic pain patients do not find a good solution to their illness using conventional approaches to pain management, Wallis concludes. And finding a "good" solution does not mean being pain free, or free from adverse drug effects.

Since it was the most helpful treatment in my case, I was glad to see Jane Brody discuss prolotherapy and explain why prolotherapy "kick-starts" tissue repair.[3] Brody notes that prolotherapy is now the subject of a controlled clinical trial sponsored by the National Center for Complementary and Alternative Medicine, part of the National Institutes of Health.

While a major breakthrough in pain research and pharmaceutical solutions cannot be ruled out, many health-care professionals point to the multidisciplinary clinic with an emphasis on alternatives as the best way to proceed. Unfortunately, much in pain management has worked against a multidisciplinary approach: the belief that only highly controlled quantitative studies can yield valid data; the inadequate and narrow training doctors traditionally have received in understanding chronic pain; health-care systems that enforce drastically brief face time with doctors; the difficulty many doctors have in dealing with suffering; the high cost of multidisciplinary clinics; and the insurance industry's aversion to alternative therapies. Scott Fishman told Wallis that insurance companies would rather pay him $1,000 to do a twenty-minute visit with an injection of chemical substances than pay him a fraction of that to spend an hour listening and talking with a patient.[4] Yet pain physicians need the time to take an extensive history, listen to the patient's story and her/his suffering, talk about living and working conditions that impact on pain, explore alternatives, and decide which other health professionals may be called for. As chronic pain patterns often change over time, this needs to be an ongoing conversation.

Claudia Wallis reports that there are fewer than two hundred multidisciplinary pain clinics in the United States. This amounts to 250,000 patients for every clinic, using a 50 million figure for people living with chronic pain and all of them having access to the two hundred clinics. Many clinics receive hundreds of referrals a month that they cannot handle. Ronald Libby, a policy analyst at the University of North Florida estimates there is one pain specialist in the United States for every six thousand pain patients who actively seek help.[5] A 2007 roundtable discussion of leading pain experts convened by the American Pain Foundation cites the figure of one pain specialist for every 21,000 pain patients.[6] In Canada, a 2006 listing of publicly funded pain clinics shows that several provinces (Prince Edward Island, Nunavit, the Yukon Territories) have none at all, while other provinces (Manitoba and Newfoundland) have only one each.[7] In the provinces that do have clinics, the average wait varies from fourteen to forty-two months. Even in the best of clinics, however, patients rarely get cured. Pain specialists prefer to talk in terms of "reducing" or "managing" pain or getting "patients back to a reasonable life from no life."[8]

The work I had to do to find ways to diminish my devilish pain required much persistence, patience, and trust. I had to believe that with careful observation of pain patterns and with steadfast engagement in a range of mind-body practices, I would be able to minimize the pain signals. I had to pursue all possibilities for treatments and explore many alternatives. I had to carefully attend to all aspects of my general health. I had to learn about drugs' adverse effects, and try to decide what misery I was willing to endure and what risks I was willing to take. I had to learn to quiet my mind to give the pain the relaxed yet alert attention that helps to decrease pain levels. I have had to learn to be vigilant to the nature of social settings and assertive enough to leave immediately when certain stimuli trigger the warning signs for pain—or signal to a visitor that I need to be alone. I have had to learn to accept the inability of others to understand my invisible disease, yet persist in trying to put them in the picture. I have had to learn the difference between healing and being cured. And though the pain itself may never be resolved, the maddening chaos it brought has subsided. Having said that, I am still a split person. A bit crazed from waking up to pain almost every morning, morphing into an often exhausted but more normal person later in the day.

Writing this book has been both difficult and therapeutic. The most difficult parts—the descriptions of the pain, the disintegration of the self, the suicidal years, the loss of friends, the seemingly uncaring doctors—served as material to work through in therapy. Reading my despair to someone I trust turned out to be deeply healing. But I dragged the pages to my therapy sessions for many weeks before I could actually read them aloud. When I finally thought I was ready to do so, I found I couldn't get through the first paragraph. Trauma imprints itself deeply on the nervous system. The rereading and rewriting of this book during the editing process has been as difficult as the original writing of it. But persisting with both has invited some order back into my life, and, bit by bit, it has brought a certain release from trauma. Borrowing Dionne Brand's words, I have tried to write this thing calmly even as its lines burn to a close.[9] The calmness I had to ascend to in order to put this book together has resembled the state of unhurried, unfragmented consciousness I have had to struggle to bring to the pain.

Not everyone, of course, wants to write. But it doesn't matter in what way one engages the processes of attention and release, of *slowing down* the habitual reactions of panic, as long as expression of the trauma is accomplished as many times as it takes for it to be exposed, thinned, and, as much as possible, dissolved.

Though the worst in terms of pain intensity, frequency, and duration is over, at least for now—nothing is ever certain when it comes to chronic pain—Wallis's words still cause my emotions to explode:

Chronic pain is a thief. It breaks into your body and robs you blind. With lightening fingers, it can take away your livelihood, your marriage, your friends, your favorite pastimes and big chunks of your personality. Left unapprehended, it will steal your days and your nights until the world has collapsed into a cramped cell of suffering.[10]

Meanwhile, for months and months, your doctor may be juggling the more than fifty drugs now available, trying to find the "right" one. But for too many of us there is no "right" drug. As it stands, chronic pain is not often an illness to be cured by doctors alone and by the pharmaceuticals they prescribe, however necessary these are. Chronic pain is a multifaceted condition woven tightly into day-to-day life, asking for multifaceted understandings and multifaceted approaches. For that we need many people.

It is not an easy task. For instance, a 2005 survey carried out for the Canadian Pain Coalition found that only 47 percent of Canadians believe that chronic pain is real.[11] Believing those who suffer from it continues to be a problem. James Henry stresses, as I do, the profound problem posed by the invisibility of the disease: "The public will ask, where are all these people?"[12] They are at home, he says: "They can't go to school or to work. There are all kinds of reasons why pain doesn't have a face." It was exciting for me to read that Henry, as the scientific director of the Michael G. DeGroote Institute for Pain Research and Care, is seeking funding to set up a nationwide ambassador program that recruits chronic pain patients into the process of understanding and treating chronic pain. Finally—a scientist is actively seeking us out as a source of information.

One of my hopes for this book then is that it will make believers out of disbelievers. I hope the reader has come to see that chronic pain is as serious an illness as cancer or heart disease. It is a different disease, and although it doesn't directly kill you, it can drive you mad.

We need an ethics of pain, both within medicine and in the larger community. This can happen only if those who are not in pain accept the claim that chronic pain makes on us all. Such empathy does not often come naturally. The instinct to turn away from others' pain is strong. Empathy asks for a deliberate ethical stance that desires to imagine the other's pain, to listen, to be present. For that, a human being needs an "ethics of listening," to borrow Arthur Frank's words.[13] An ethics of listening that leads to an ethics of being.

In June 2005 Congressman Michael Rogers of Michigan held hearings in which he invited chronic pain patients to testify about their pain management—or lack thereof—to raise public and political awareness, and I wish I could have been there to read from my story.[14] While an estimated 50 to 90 million people in North America live in chronic pain, says Rogers, the National Institutes of Health spends less than 1 percent of its research budget on all types of pain. Chronic pain is draining the economy of billions of dollars, yet federal agencies are doing little if anything about it, he adds.

Further efforts by Michael Rogers, Congresswoman Lois Capps of California, the American Pain Foundation, and over one hundred partnering pain and pain–advocacy organizations resulted on September 24, 2008, in the passing of the National Pain Care Policy Act of 2008 (HR 2994) by the U.S. House of Representatives. This legislation authorizes the convening of an Institute of Medicine conference on pain care, creating an interagency committee to identify gaps in pain research, expanding collaboration in pain research across federal agencies and the private sector, and providing the means to improve health professionals' understanding and ability to assess and treat pain. It further requires the secretary of health and human services to develop and implement a national educational outreach and awareness campaign on pain as a public health problem.

As I near the completion of this book, I feel relief in knowing that this important legislation is on its way to the U.S. Senate for approval and I cannot imagine that senators representing millions of people in pain would not pass it. They better. Then, the hard work will continue. The hard work of addressing the details of this broad legislative outline. The hard work of convincing all the various communities involved that chronic pain, while intensely personal, is not just a personal or a medical story. That pain lives and breathes among us. That pain belongs to all of us and that ignoring pain is no longer an option.

Clinical Commentary

Scott M. Fishman, MD

I have been working in the field of pain medicine for many years and have cared for thousands of patients. While no two patients' experiences are the same, I have heard innumerable stories that highlight the central dilemma of this book: that, for many patients like Lous Heshusius, the health-care system itself is a major source of pain and suffering. In the story presented by Heshusius, the patient suffers from chronic pain, but as she struggles toward recovery, her central problem is compounded by a maze of clinicians, contradictory information and advice, and adversarial bureaucracy. As she sometimes successfully—often unsuccessfully—navigates this maze, her pain, which started in her neck, invades her entire life and undermines her quality of life.

Experiences like those of Lous Heshusius are the result, in part, of the reductionist nature of our health-care system, in which the focus is on dissecting people and disease down to the smallest possible objective elements—detecting a molecule in the blood, capturing an image, illuminating receptors, visualizing cells, determining an immune footprint, or searching for some other small but incontrovertible finding in support of the ultimate cause of the disease that troubles a patient. Once it determines the cause, then the system focuses on reversing that cause and thus curing the disease.

Unfortunately, pain is neither a single disease entity nor a testable hypothesis. Pain simply can't be proved or disproved. In a medical world more committed to solving the crime than comforting the afflicted, the individual in pain confronts a system that has wandered far from its fundamental promise to patients of curing when we can but always treating suffering.

We do this because of our incomplete understanding of pain. Most of us think of pain as a sensation or a perception of a noxious stimulus. Pain is the alarm system in the human body that tells us about imminent harm, actual harm, or healing. That alarm system is connected to measurable biological and physiological responses that are associated with distinct molecules and cells in the body. However, that is not all that is involved in pain. Pain is a multidimensional phenomenon that integrates perception with emotion to form the complex experience of suffering. Although you may be able to identify a precipitating event, the end result is like a symphony in which you are able to hear the themes but unable to distinguish all of the many instruments.

When someone is in pain, her or his mind and body are inextricably linked and there is at least some degree of suffering. Indeed, a critical question to address is: If the pain doesn't cause suffering, is it pain? The answer isn't entirely clear. Without the suffering, what we might call pain is essentially noxious sensation. And when we are suffering in ways that do not involve pain, we know that any painful sensation is experienced more intensely. Although we have learned a great deal from neuroscience about how pain is processed, this valuable yet reductionist knowledge does not inform us about the greater scope of how it produces suffering, which too often undermines all domains of a person's quality of life. We can't be satisfied with simply understanding how the parts work. In a December 16, 2001, article in the *New York Times Magazine* by Melanie Thernstrom, Dr. Daniel Carr, the Saltonstall Professor of Pain Research at Tufts University in Boston, compared pain and its sensations with time and a clock. You can know all the parts of a clock, he noted, but that isn't time.

Although we are learning more and more about the mechanics of pain, the suffering associated with it is more elusive. The experience of suffering is informed by everything in our lives, including the emotional, spiritual, and social aspects that physicians too often feel unprepared to encounter. Because of this, suffering patients may feel abandoned, left playing what may seem to them to be a shell game in which they are disadvantaged, with little control and few options. The complex mind-body dimension of their disorder not only speaks directly to the frailty of the human condition but also points to the potential for inhumanity within medicine.

In my practice, for example, patients are often very worried that we're going to tell them that the pain they experience is "all in their head." I think these patients are really afraid that we will ignore or dismiss the problem that they are concerned about and, in its place, give them a stigmatizing diagnosis. They don't want to be told that they have a mental rather than a physical illness. By giving them an explanation or diagnosis that even hints that there may be a mental process involved, they fear that the physical basis of their ailment will be denied. More than this they may be concerned that the people on whom they depend for help will relinquish the responsibility to get them better.

Early in my career, when I talked to patients I tried to be as clear as possible that I believed that their pain was physical and that I would not attribute problems I didn't understand to being all in their head. I didn't want to tell patients that there was any emotional component to their problem because I didn't want them to feel judged, stigmatized, and diminished. But ultimately I came to my senses as I recognized a very simple concept— you can't have pain without a head. By disregarding the mind's contribution to chronic pain, one does not do justice to the patient. So now I say to patients, "I'm sorry, but you can't have pain without a head. Pain is in your head to some degree. But that doesn't mean I believe it's not in your body. It doesn't mean your pain is not physical." Ultimately, I have come to see pain as challenging those of us in Western medicine to take a holistic view of patients. We must literally view a whole person that includes a mind and a body together.

Unfortunately, as this book so well describes, medicine's reductionist focus fragments the clinical gaze and gives us a fractured view of, and approach to, our patients. It has been said that too often today doctors have relationships with diseases rather than patients. Quite frankly, when someone is suffering with something we don't understand, it may be much easier for a physician to relate to the diagnosis, or lack thereof, than to the person. But this leads to an exacerbation of the kind of suffering the author experienced. Why wasn't there one person who was invested in all aspects of Ms. Heshusius's care? Why did this patient have to go searching from one doctor to the next only to find that each doctor took responsibility for only a part of the problem? The answer is that her experience stems from the way we approach pain care in the United States, Canada, and in too many other parts of the world.

By focusing on and reducing our gaze to disease, and fragmenting patients into a series of diseases, medicine has simplified what would otherwise be an overwhelmingly complex set of human phenomena and experiences. Because of this reductionist approach, we have, in fact, cured many diseases. Our success helps to explain why in the United States and throughout the industrialized world, eighty to ninety year olds are the fastest growing segment of our population. Yet, statistics suggest that in the United States many people in older age groups have chronic pain. The question that must therefore be raised is, are these people living longer and living well, or are they living longer only to suffer more?

To answer that question we must understand that medical fragmentation can victimize a patient like Lous Heshusius. The medical system becomes a labyrinth, and as a patient's condition becomes increasingly complex and difficult to treat, there are proportionately fewer committed guides. Most often, patients are left to navigate for themselves as best they can. In this story we have a very intelligent patient who's resourceful and capable—and look at how she struggled, how incapacitated and disabled she became—trying to figure out how to get through this maze. Imagine how someone with fewer resources would fare? So the system compounds the pain because it doesn't offer an integrated model for approaching this amorphous condition of being in chronic pain. We don't have a model that is able to first see the whole person and then coordinate their care.

It has been difficult to develop such a model because pain medicine—which is a multidisciplinary field, comprising clinicians from fields ranging from psychology to surgery, alternative to conventional medicine, and from care of newborns to patients at the end of life—is practiced as a subspecialty with no appropriate primary discipline to call home. Within the most conventional boundaries of our discipline we might have anesthesiologists, physical medicine and rehabilitation specialists, psychiatrists, internists, and neurologists. All call themselves pain doctors. But none of us is fully trained to integrate everything that we need to know. In contrast, if you look at, say, a cardiologist, you find he or she starts off as an internal medicine doctor and then focuses on the heart. It makes sense to learn about the medical issues of the whole body and then specialize. There is no such process for pain medicine, and that's what Ms. Heshusius confronted. She very poignantly tells the story of how she went from one specialist to another. Each one thought they might be of help but didn't have the tools to pull it all together.

It's important for clinicians to understand what can happen to a patient who is confronted with this kind of medical fragmentation. The danger is that, as with Lous Heshusius, what started out as a focal disorder can take over a patient's whole life. Down the line there was not only the primary problem but all sorts of collateral damage with which she had to deal. Like many patients, what came first, which led to what came next, became less important than how a body part in pain spread to and created a life in pain. This then robbed the patient of quality in all domains of her life. The complexity of the problem was reflected in the difficulty of integrating potential solutions.

In this case, and so many others, instead of finding an integrative solution, the clinical approach was to watch and wait. This attitude that we won't treat the pain aggressively now but will watch and see how it develops characterized the view of many of the physicians Heshusius encountered on her journey.

Many physicians believed—and still believe—that this kind of watching and waiting does not have any negative consequences for patients. They believe that not treating pain is the safest thing they can do both for patients and themselves. Fortunately, many in medicine have begun to understand that when someone is in pain there's no risk-free option—including doing nothing. But too many doctors still allow patients to be in pain while they wait and see how things are going to evolve. Even though we know that such an approach negatively affects patients and can even be lethal, some doctors still allow a patient to languish in pain, believing that, on balance, such an experience isn't detrimental to the patient's health and well being.

They do this for many reasons. Medical decisions are always based on weighing risk against benefit. Doing nothing may be the best thing if the treatment choices are potentially more harmful. However, this has to be weighed against the possible harm associated with doing nothing. If doing nothing is the least risky option, that's what we do, whether we are dealing with pain or anything else. After all, a fundamental philosophy in medicine is "first do no harm." The key question is, is doing nothing doing no harm? In medical education and medical practice we must recognize that allowing someone to remain in pain has risks. But doctors have not been taught that pain—in and of itself—adds weight to the risk-benefit calculation. We must understand that there is usually something, if not many things, we can do when someone is in pain that has less risk than allowing them to remain in pain. And we must understand that there are always things we can do.

I have a saying that "we can't cure everyone, but we can make almost everyone better." This means that although we may not be able to cure or reverse the underlying problem, there is usually a lot we can do to improve quality of life.

When we choose not to treat someone in pain, it often says more about us, as clinicians, than it says about our patients. It says something about our fear. It says something about our knowledge base. It says something about our willingness to take risks. Perhaps we're afraid to produce an addict or drug-seeker or abuser. Or it may mean that we have made a judgment and believe the patient's pain isn't real and we would be enabling them if we treated them. Or it may mean we don't have the comprehensive knowledge that gives us enough confidence to take a particular step that would be required to treat pain.

The unfortunate reality is that very few doctors are taught much about pain. They're not taught about how pain works, nor are they taught much about how the alarm system of pain can be broken. Doctors aren't taught enough about rational and safe use of analgesic drugs or other pain-relieving treatments. And as the pendulum has swung from minimal awareness of the need for pain control to much wider acceptance or even demand for it, the average doctor now feels that there is an obligation to treat—but they feel very uncomfortable because they are largely not confident about how to do it. So this creates a vicious cycle for patients and clinicians alike.

Patients who are trapped in this vicious cycle are easily labeled. We say the patient is "amplifying" because they're angry or frustrated. Or maybe we say they have a "personality disorder." In fact anyone who is stressed enough will look like they have a personality disorder. Then we blame the patient. We call them a crock and they call us a quack.

This kind of cycle of blame is inevitable when doctors aren't prepared to adequately manage a patient's pain. Without the education and tools needed to manage pain, doctors feel imperfect and thus uncomfortable. Physicians—who consider themselves to be men and women of science—feel particularly vulnerable when they lack the tools necessary to do their jobs. When people feel uncomfortable and vulnerable because they don't know what to do, they may either blame themselves or blame the "customer." It is only human nature. And sadly because pain elicits so many emotional reactions, it's not hard to find a reason to blame that customer, which happens time and time again. That's why patients feel we are stigmatizing them by labeling them as either "nuts" or as seeking "secondary gain."

Let's consider this latter case. Clinicians often claim that patients continue to have symptoms because they are getting some sort of "secondary gain" from their complaints. The classic case is a patient who is suffering from pain while seeking workers' compensation for their work-related injury. This is the patient who is often labeled as having lost their amateur status. Unfortunately, this concept of "secondary gain" is not widely or well understood. What does secondary gain mean? It means that the person has an unstated reason for doing what they're doing that isn't being directly dealt with in the examination room. Of course, that sometimes happens. The scientific literature shows, however, that we're not very good at determining who has this undermining type of agenda, because the reality is that everyone has some secondary gain agenda.

This is why, when we are tempted to label someone as having a secondary gain agenda, we have to think very carefully. We all seek secondary gains from the things we do. We want all sorts of things for all sorts of complicated reasons. Doctors aren't exempt from this. What defines the doctor in the therapeutic role is that we are supposed to be solely focused on the best care of the patient. So our primary gain may be to help the person. But there are many other secondary gain agendas. For example, we're getting paid for our services. And doctors are certainly guilty of being focused on reimbursement.

Doctors are often shocked to learn that there is, in fact, a literature that documents the negative impact of labeling a patient as seeking secondary gain. This data reveals that there is, in fact, a phenomenon called "professional secondary gain." By labeling a patient, the person treating the patient as having a secondary gain agenda, asserts his or her belief that the patient's primary complaint isn't valid and that the patient is essentially a fake. Taking such a position makes it easy for the clinician to relinquish responsibility to get the patient better. So when we label the patient it may say more about us than them.

If doctors don't have the tools needed to deal with chronic pain, they may display the kind of negative attitudes that Heshusius describes. Many of the clinicians she encountered seemed to deliberately deny her any hint of hope. This highlights another of the dilemmas we face as physicians. On the one hand, we always want to use the positive impact of hope. We know that faith and hope have healing power and that they can be enormously beneficial. On the other hand, we don't want to give false hope, and we certainly don't want to enable patients to harm themselves by being unrealistic. The key, for us, as clinicians, is to ask ourselves what do we know and what don't we know and to be very careful about what we don't know.

As I said before, I tell my patients that I can't cure everyone but I can make almost everyone better. It just depends on how you define "better." When you're looking at chronic pain, as this book reflects and I think this patient would agree, part of her body was in pain and this created a life in pain, which in turn led to all sorts of collateral losses. Even though a clinician might not be able to have an impact on the primary sense of pain, we could help to improve other areas of her quality of life that have been amplifying her suffering and dampening her hope of a positive future.

Even though I may not agree with what I might believe to be an overly optimistic view or unrealistic expectations, I'm rarely pessimistic. The only time I'm consistently pessimistic is when my patient is pessimistic and unwilling to be involved in his or her own care. For example, this may occur in a patient who comes to me asking for help yet conveys the impression that not only I, the doctor, will fail but that he or she, the patient, will not be part of the solution. When that happens, I have to be pessimistic. I usually explain that medicine can only do so much. We're not the scientists that we're purported to be and we're not the technological whiz-bang problem solvers we have represented ourselves to be. In fact, medicine is an art, and all that I can do is be a counselor and a coach while the patient runs the race. My potential as a clinician is proportional to the patient's willingness to be a partner.

Similarly, a patient's potential for improved quality of life can be dependent on a physician's willingness to partner, to say, "I will go through this journey with you, and I will be your consultant." This is something only one physician that Ms. Heshusius talked with seemed willing to say. Yet this is the way medicine should work. Ideally, physicians should avoid paternalistic and inappropriate roles such as that of parent, priest, or boss. We physicians are consultants who can offer expert knowledge and experience. But the patient is the decision maker. We need to walk through this journey with them and offer them every reasonable option possible. In my practice, for example, anything that is safe is in play. Period. It doesn't matter what it is, whether I agree with it or not. If it's safe, it's okay. The only time I will say, "I don't want you to do something" is if I think that it's going to produce more harm than good. And once the options are clear, I always remember that the final decision is the patient's.

Treating pain involves all sorts of different modalities. In this book, the author talks about prolotherapy, meditation, and psychotherapy. Other people find relief from acupuncture or many other disparate techniques—some of which physicians consider to be unconventional. Some physicians may resist unconventional treatments, not because we don't like them, but because we are taught to look at things that we can objectify, that have a molecular weight, can be imaged on an X-ray or MRI, or can be tested so that something turns pink or blue. You can't do that with acupuncture or a lot of other therapies. These therapies have a broad and integrated impact on life that is much like pain itself.

We need wider acceptance of the idea that when we are treating patients in pain anything that's safe and effective is in play. With many therapies, I don't need to know why they're effective, and, unfortunately, all too often I don't. Let's take acupuncture, which is something that's been very effective for some of my patients and doesn't work at all for others. The key is to be very honest about my being unable to predict for whom it will work. I can take one patient and send him to ten different acupuncturists and I get ten different treatments for the same problem. Yet acupuncture is the most time-tested therapy in medicine. Research clearly demonstrates its effectiveness, and, unlike many other options, it has minimal risks. So, in terms of safety, it's a no-brainer. But I still can't say how it works or exactly what it does, and that makes me as a doctor very uncomfortable.

Alternatively, there are many therapies that can do both good and harm. As physicians we face weighing and balancing risk versus benefit in all medical decisions. Prolotherapy, which helped Lous Heshusius, is a good example. Some doctors don't like it because they don't understand it. Some doctors who don't like it do understand it and are worried about its potential and unknown negative consequences. I can fully appreciate that an individual would say, "I understand the risks and I want to take the risk." I think we, as physicians, must be able to work within this admittedly imperfect system and commit to serving the patient in helping her make a choice.

Patients in chronic pain run the same kind of marathon as elite athletes, which is why it's useful to consider the insights of sports psychology when dealing with patients in pain. Let's say Lance Armstrong is crimping out at that last hill of the Tour de France. He is feeling pain and his brain is screaming out, "Stop! Enough! Slow down! Quit!" Our patients are essentially running the same marathon, and the skills that Lance Armstrong uses can be used in their everyday lives to give them the needed endurance and ability to perform. What are these skills? They are the same skills Buddhists have known about for thousands of years. They are skills that help us to control what's in the scope of our consciousness and select what is fully, partially, and not in our attention. By doing this we can help patients gain control over the pain they once thought enslaved them.

These skills are not a global cure but rather a source of vital control that allows for reengagement with the parts of life that have been incapacitated and that led to the substantial collateral losses that eroded quality of life. If, for a period of time of your choosing, you can focus away from your pain, you can have a relationship with a friend, perform a task, or simply relax without the attention-devouring impact of the pain. Now you may be able to regain lost aspects of your social life, or reach back into your marriage, or interact with your children, or return to your church. And there are many different varieties of techniques that can be employed.

I find that most patients are open to some of these tools and not to others. We have to tailor them for what works for the person. Lance Armstrong isn't going to use the same tools as Michael Jordan. It's all individual, and fortunately there are many different tools and combinations to choose from.

As the author's daughter illustrates in this book, family members and friends can be a vital part of the toolkit that patients mobilize to deal with their pain. They are significant assets. Unfortunately, as chronic pain sets in and all aspects of life become increasingly challenging, many patients feel they lose their friends rather than incorporate them into the solution. It's a balancing act for people in pain because their suffering is not well tolerated. All you have to do is go to the oncology floor of any hospital to see this firsthand. There aren't as many visitors. Missing are the candy stripers and other cheerful volunteers. It's naturally uncomfortable for people who aren't suffering to be in that space. So maintaining social connections is a challenge. The collateral impact of chronic pain is physical and psychological as well as social and spiritual, which means that mind-body work is required for recovery.

As we've seen throughout this story, doctors and other clinicians, family members and friends all have an impact on a patient who suffers from chronic pain. As the author points out, insurers and government regulators also have a tremendous influence on the outcome of such a marathon. Both of these groups reflect the narrow, fragmented vision that is embedded not only in contemporary clinical practice but in how that practice is reimbursed and regulated.

Consider reimbursement. Today, a managed-care insurance company would much rather pay me $1,000 or more to spend ten minutes with a patient to give her an injection in the spine than spend an hour with a patient like Lous Heshusius figuring out which kind of treatments are best for her. The insurer will balk at that, make me fill out papers, make me make telephone calls to toll-free numbers and defend myself after a compulsory period of waiting on hold. On the other hand, they will immediately, with no questions asked, accept my charges if I do the standard procedure. Although it would cost far less to spend the hour with a patient and their family, the reductionist model of medicine ironically assures that potentially less effective—but also more costly—treatments may be offered.

Why? Because insurance companies believe they can patrol such treatment. The insurance company says, "I know he used a needle, he used a drug, he has images to show what he did, and I know exactly how the procedure is performed. It's all objective, therefore we will pay for it." But they don't know what to make of the hour I spend with a patient and his or her family. How do they know what happened during that hour? How do they know I did what I said I did? How do they understand what I did?

Although paying for ineffective and costly treatment may seem irrational, such irrationality is rampant throughout the financial structure of the health-care system.

When it comes to pain, regulation may be equally irrational. For example, in Washington state the government is responding to the problem of rising prescription drug abuse. The Medicaid and workers' compensation branch of the state government has come up with guidelines for physicians. They suggest that physicians who prescribe more than a certain amount of an opioid pain reliever (such as morphine-type medications) should get a pain specialist involved. Washington state regulators, however, neither define what a specialist is nor consider how to pay for this additional consultation, which is expensive. Doctors are likely to believe that if they can't get a specialist, which, given the scarcity of pain specialists, they know they will have difficulty doing, then they are going to be looked at as substandard. So they may think, why get involved? why even start?

Society is clearly saying—and rightfully so—that we've got a public health crisis of undertreated pain. Patients are demanding care, and doctors are being pushed to the frontline of this problem. But doctors are also getting mixed messages. Society is telling them they have to manage pain even though they're not trained to do it. Many doctors who don't feel competent will avoid treating pain patients at all. Some of them do treat such patients but don't know how to do it appropriately. And if they don't do it appropriately, the regulators come up with regulations that make things even more difficult. It's a maladaptive and vicious cycle.

This cycle is being challenged in specific areas of medicine such as in treatment of back pain and expensive back surgeries. In some regions of the United States, back surgery is far more common than in others, but the outcomes, both in health and cost have not improved. The cost to society is astronomical, and the benefit is questionable. We talk to state bureaucrats and say, "This is crazy. If you would have paid for the appropriate care of the patient in the first place, you wouldn't have had to pay for the back surgery or for all the costly problems that ensued when it didn't work." It may have cost more in the beginning, but the value can be seen over time.

On the other hand, the one area in the care of chronic pain that's absolutely proven to work is the multidisciplinary rehabilitative model that would have helped the author of this book early on. But you can't often get it paid for because it's relatively expensive in the short run, and insurance payers see it as a black hole of reimbursement. Like talking with patients, it is hard to definitively prove that there is a positive financial or clinical outcome—until, that is, we discover how much doing nothing or making fragmented treatment decisions really costs. But at that point, much therapeutic opportunity may be lost, and much unnecessary damage may have occurred. Fortunately, many are focusing on the global cost and negative impact of the treatments. The tendency for insurance companies to pay for expensive procedures, for which they know the exact breakdown of costs, is increasingly being questioned both from health and economic perspectives. Likewise, investment of multidisciplinary resources, both preventively and early on in the course of disease, is increasingly being recognized as good medical and economic practice.

It seems that to make a real difference in this misguided cycle of care, we must start at the beginning and make the commitment to educate our medical students and doctors about how to appropriately manage pain. Medicine also has to prioritize pain relief as a positive outcome in itself by changing its fragmented and compartmentalized structure so that clinicians can integrate the breadth of knowledge and disparate resources necessary to improve quality of life. If medicine leads the way, insurers and regulators may follow, which is why education is so crucial.

Pain is the most common reason a patient seeks medical care, yet medical students are barely taught pain management, let alone a holistic (not alternative) view of the patient as a person with a disease. This disease is no different than other chronic illnesses, and in many ways it may lead to greater devastation. The only way to effectively deal with chronic pain is to reconsider how we train doctors, nurses, and clinicians of all kinds, including physical therapists, pharmacists, and so on. We must start to recognize that we've reached diminishing returns with the reductionist model of you cure, cure, cure, and then when you fail, you treat for comfort. We have very good data that show that we can both cure and comfort at the same time and that, when we do, we see improved results in terms of overall health and quality of life. We can look at people as whole people rather than just as embodiments of diseases. It's clearly more humanistic. Perhaps it's more time consuming to work that way, but overall it will be more effective and less expensive. The cost to society of pursuing ineffective diagnostic workups and treatments is enormous. Moreover, the cost in suffering is immeasurable.

As Ms. Heshusius found, there was no single individual who would or could serve as the central manager to integrate the disparate disciplines needed for her as a patient. Because of this, her journey required dozens of clinicians, tests, and treatments—all without much benefit. Like those she encountered, the average neurologist may not be considering the impact of joint arthritis from disuse. The rheumatologist may miss the early nerve damage, while the physiatrist may focus on physical therapy but fail to notice that the patient's insomnia and depression are driving a downward cycle of dysfunction. Each clinician brought their special keyhole perspective through which they added on but did not integrate and incorporate a global view or approach to her treatment.

Recognizing the impact of the failure to treat the whole patient with a global approach will push change. This global approach must recognize the shortcomings of a fragmented model that assigns each patient and problem to a primary discipline based on specific disease pathologies, organ parts, or the place in which care is delivered. This model doesn't recognize that the prevalence of suffering is interwoven throughout the patient's experience. Because of this, none of the primary fields take ownership of symptom management or suffering. This needs to change.

As I said before, pain medicine is a subspecialty that has no primary discipline; pain care, symptom management, and dealing with suffering is an orphan within major medicine. It's an orphan within the National Institutes of Health in the United States and in other countries where it also has no home. It has inadequately organized forces to fight for it. Therefore, it's too often an afterthought. Pain and symptom management is underfunded relative to other disorders in the NIH in the United States, even though pain is the most common reason for consulting a doctor. This underfunding parallels the fact that we don't teach medical students about pain and symptom management, which, in turn, guarantees that doctors will feel uncomfortable treating chronic pain, which leads to inadequate or inappropriate treatment. It's one common thread through this whole fabric.

To weave an entirely different kind of cloth, we need national and international recognition in all our health-care systems that curing and improving quality of life are equal goals. We need to offer care that is not solely focused on the patient saying, "I feel better" but is fundamentally invested in the patient functionally *being* better. Because there's no one field that focuses on quality of life and assures that medicine is doing what it can across the life spectrum and across all of its other disciplines, it's time that the medical field recognizes its responsibility and reorganizes itself for the greater good of patients and society. Continuing down our current path is undermining the care that people receive and adding substantial economic burden to society.

To create a new model of care in the United States, a number of players would need to be involved. These include the Liaison Committee on Medical Education (the organization that accredits medical schools), the American Council on Graduate Medical Education (the organization that accredits medical internships and residency training programs), the American Board of Medical Specialties (the board that certifies physicians), and the American Medical Association (the organization that represents practicing physicians). These groups need to agree to define an area of medicine that focuses on quality of life and that would include the area that I work in that's connected to pain, symptom management, and suffering throughout the life span.

There is a real need to correct the current situation in which separate disciplines overlap with each other but have no integrating structure. For example, in many hospitals there are actually two pain services, one for patients who aren't dying (Pain Medicine) and one for patients who are (Palliative Medicine). Yet everything we do in pain medicine is essentially palliative care, except we usually don't discriminate against people who aren't dying. And although there are certainly differences between treating suffering at the end of life and the suffering of chronic disease, the overlap is substantial. It is counterproductive to develop clinicians who are unable to intervene at any given point on the continuum of pain and suffering. In order to produce physicians who have the skill to effectively treat pain we need to create a home within medicine for all of the subdisciplines that diagnose and treat pain and suffering. These include acute pain management, chronic pain management, pediatric pain management, interventional pain management, rehabilitative pain care, psychological pain care, and palliative care.

If we recall how the primary discipline of Emergency Medicine was created, this will provide us with an excellent model. Before the late 1960s, hospital emergency rooms were staffed by hospital physicians who were trained in a single discipline such as general surgery, psychiatry, dermatology, internal medicine, who rotated through the ER on an episodic basis. No single physician was invested in the comprehensive journey a patient was taking during an emergency. The surgeon would focus on his part, and the internist, radiologist, pediatrician, and cardiologist would focus on theirs. No one was trained with the comprehensive knowledge that would be needed to handle the full breadth of an emergency.

Physicians who worked in the emergency room recognized the limitations of this fragmented model. They decided to leave their particular single practices and join together to form a new specialty. In 1968 a group of such pioneering physicians founded the American College of Emergency Physicians, and in 1970 Cincinnati General Hospital established the first Emergency Medicine residency training program. Once the ACEP was established, the American Medical Association recognized emergency medicine training programs, and in 1979, the American Board of Medical Specialties voted to recognize Emergency Medicine as a recognized specialty. Today, thirty-eight years later, Emergency Medicine is an established discipline in and of itself, with its own home, its own training programs, and no hospital emergency department would consider operating without Emergency Medicine specialists.

To create a new primary specialty that deals with pain and quality of life that, like Emergency Medicine, does not focus on a disease or part of the body that's diseased, will not be easy. It will not happen overnight and will take a lot of work and energy, particularly if our goal is to create a discipline that is integrative and that does not isolate itself in yet another medical silo. Many of us are working toward this solution, but for pain patients and their clinicians, the end goal is not entirely in sight.

This means that patients who need immediate care will be best served by appreciating the limitations of their health-care system and compensating by increasing their knowledge and self-advocacy. Long gone are the days when health-care systems reliably pulled it all together for their patients. Today, medical care is viewed as a product and patients are all too often viewed as customers. In this market model, the buyer must beware. To effectively navigate the system, individuals need to become knowledgeable about how it works. Yet many people spend more time and energy educating themselves about the cars they buy than the health care they get. I suspect many feel that participating in their own health care is futile, that it may be too complicated or even inappropriate to do so. In many ways, the science of medicine has reinforced this through the doctor-knows-best attitude of the past.

As articulated throughout this book, self-advocacy—requiring knowledge about the disease as well as about how to navigate the system—is essential. Few can run this marathon alone, and the alternative is feeling isolated and abandoned. On the other hand, there are so many resources out there that the landscape can seem daunting if not frightening. Although patients must become informed, they must choose their information carefully. They must also choose their clinicians carefully and be open to as broad an array of potential solutions as possible, not settling for inadequate care. Typically, the primary-care physician is the first stop, but in the absence of clear and convincing results, moving on to other clinicians with more to offer is not only appropriate but often necessary for making timely progress. Determining exactly whom to go to next may require research and consideration that may not be obtainable from the patient's primary-care or specialty clinicians. Therefore, patients and their loved ones are left to take on this unexpected role. Help is out there and books like those listed in the resource section of this text make for a good first stop. Consumer organizations such as the American Pain Foundation (www.painfoundation.org) can provide a wide array of information and connect individuals who have common problems or needs. Above all, no one should be left to suffer alone.

I hope that patients—and those clinicians, families, and friends who share their lives and their journey—will seriously reflect on the insights that Lous Heshusius has shared. If they combine this with other available information, they may be able to enter any level of the health system as their own best advocate. I am also hopeful we can unite in our common need to make substantive changes in both medicine and society so that anyone suffering and in pain can find the financial and clinical resources as well as the human compassion necessary to make an immediate difference.

I continue to feel very hopeful that we can expect to achieve major advances in the treatment of pain in the near future. I believe we will develop new paradigms that will more effectively counter the destructive effects of pain throughout the body and mind. This will involve advancing the best of technology as well as our current understanding of the molecular and cellular organization of the human being. Yet, even as we bring further understanding to the pieces that make us up, I believe we will further recognize the miraculous complexity of the whole person. I hope we can remain open to the many mysteries and possibilities of how we work and how we may help ourselves to heal.

Resource Guide

To Find a Pain Specialist

American Academy of Family Physicians
www.familydoctor.org

American Academy of Nurse Practitioners
www.aanp.org
202-966-6414

American Academy of Pain Management
www.aapainmanage.org
209-533-9744

American Academy of Pain Medicine
www.painmed.org
847-375-4731

American Academy of Physician Assistants
www.aapa.org
703-836-2272

American Board of Pain Medicine
www.abpm.org
847-375-4726

American Medical Association
www.ama-assn.org
312-464-5000

American Pain Foundation
www.painfoundation.org
1-888-615-PAIN (7246)

Case Management Resource Guide
www.cmrg.com
800-784-2332

Commission on Accreditation of Rehabilitation Facilities
www.carf.org
520-325-1044

Mayo Clinic Pain Management Center
www.mayoclinic.com

National Hospice and Palliative Care Organization
www.nhpco.org
703-837-1500

National Pain Foundation
www.nationalpainfoundation.org
Pain.com
www.pain.com/painclinics/default.cfm

To Find a Complementary and Alternative Medicine Specialist

American Academy of Medical Acupuncture
www.medicalacupuncture.org
323-937-5514

American Association for Naturopathic Physicians
www.naturopathic.org
866-538-2267

American Association of Oriental Medicine
www.aaom.org
866-455-7999

American Chiropractic Association
www.amerchiro.org
703-276-8800

American Holistic Health Association
www.ahha.org
714-779-6152

American Massage Therapy Association
www.amtamassage.org
877-905-2700

American Osteopathic Association
www.osteopathic.org
800-621-1773

American Physical Therapy Association
www.apta.org
703-684-APTA (2782)

To Find a Support Group

American Chronic Pain Association
www.theacpa.org
800-533-3231

Caring Connections
www.caringinfo.org
800-658-8898

Family Caregiver Alliance
www.caregiver.org
800-445-8106

Friends' Health Connection
www.friendshealthconnection.org
800-48-FRIEND (483-7436)

National Chronic Pain Society
http://ncps-cpr.net
281-357-4673

National Family Caregivers Association
www.thefamilycaregiver.org
800-896-3650

PainAid
www.painfoundation.org

Pain Connection
www.pain-connection.org
301-309-2444

Well Spouse Association
www.wellspouse.org
800-838-0879

Resources in Canada

For professionals and researchers

Canadian Pain Society
http://www.canadianpainsoceity.ca

Canadian Pain Foundation
http://www.painfoundation.org/

Quebéc Pain Research Network
http://www.qprn.ca

For patients as well as professionals

Chronic Pain Association of Canada
http://www.chronicpaincanada.com

Association Quebecoise de la douleur chronique
http://www.douleurchronique.org

Canadian Pain Coalition
www.canadianpaincoalition.ca/

ACTION Atlantic
http://www.paincantwait.ca/

ACTION Ontario
http://www.actionontario.ca/

ACTION West
http://www.nepaction.ca

Note: The listing of resources in the United States is adapted from the American Pain Foundation's *Pain Resource Guide: Getting the Help You Need,* available on their website, www.painfoundation.org. The Canadian resources have been supplied by Lous Heshusius.

Notes

Foreword

1. Kathryn Montgomery, *How Doctors Think: Clinical Judgment and the Practice of Medicine* (New York: Oxford University Press, 2005); and Jerome E. Groopman, *How Doctors Think* (Boston: Houghton Mifflin, 2007).

2. Michael Polanyi, *Personal Knowledge: Towards a Post-Critical Philosophy,* corrected edition (Chicago: University of Chicago Press, 1962).

3. Antonio R. Damasio, *Descartes' Error: Emotion, Reason, and the Human Brain* (New York: G. P. Putnam's Sons, 1994).

4. Joan Didion, *The Year of Magical Thinking* (New York: Alfred A. Knopf, 2005).

5. David A. Williams and Francis J. Keefe, "Pain Beliefs and the Use of Cognitive-Behavioral Coping Strategies," *Pain* 46, no. 2 (1991): 185–90; Mark P. Jensen, Judith A. Turner, Joan M. Romano, and Paul Karoly, "Coping with Chronic Pain: A Critical Review of the Literature," *Pain* 47, no. 3 (1991): 249–83; Inge E. Lamé, Madelon L. Peters, Johan W. S. Vlaeyen, Maarten v. Kleef, and Jacob Patijn, "Quality of Life in Chronic Pain Is More Associated with Beliefs about Pain, Than with Pain Intensity," *European Journal of Pain* 9, no. 1 (2005): 15–24; and Steve R. Woby, Martin Urmston, and Paul J. Watson, "Self-Efficacy Mediates the Relation between Pain-Related Fear and Outcome in Chronic Low Back Pain Patients," *European Journal of Pain* 11, no. 7 (2007): 711–18.

6. R. H. Gracely, M. E. Geisser, T. Giesecke, M. A. B. Grant, F. Petzke, D. A. Williams and D. J. Clauw, "Pain Catastrophizing and Neural Responses to Pain among Persons with Fibromyalgia," *Brain* 127, no. 4 (2004): 835–43.

7. Rita Charon, "A Narrative Medicine for Pain," in *Narrative, Pain, and Suffering,* ed. Daniel B. Carr, John D. Loeser, and David B. Morris (Seattle: IASP Press, 2005), 29–44; and David B. Morris, "Narrative Medicines: Challenge and Resistance," *Permanente Journal* 12, no. 1 (2008): 88–96.

Introduction

1. Elaine Scarry, *The Body in Pain: The Making and Unmaking of the World* (New York: Oxford University Press, 1985), 9.

2. Prolotherapy consists of a series of ligament injections with a harmless substance (dextrose in my case) to bring about inflamation. The process of healing that results proliferates (hence "prolotherapy") ligament fibers, strengthening the ligaments and stabilizing the joints, relieving pain.

3. National Institute of Neurological Disorders and Stroke, January 7, 2003, http://www.ninds.nih.gov/news_events/news_articles/news_articles_chronic_pain.htm.

4. Canadian Pain Coalition, November 7, 2005, Http://www.thehealthline.ca/view news.asp?newsid=497.

5. Canadian Consortium on Pain Mechanisms Diagnosis and Management, Network Program, Final Report: Market Analysis, http://www.curepain.ca/programs.htm.

6. Report on Congressional Briefing on Pain held June 13, 2006. http://www.pain foundation.org/page.asp?file=Action/Briefing061306/BriefingReport2006.

7. David B. Morris, *The Culture of Pain* (Berkeley: University of California Press, 1991), 73–74.

8. Ibid., vi.

1. A Life Altered

1. Steven K. H. Aung, foreword to *The Treatment of Pain with Chinese Herbs and Acupuncture,* ed. Sun Peilin (New York: Churchill Livingstone, 2002), xv.

2. Michael Clark, "Managing Chronic Pain, Depression and Antidepressants: Issues and Relationships," Johns Hopkins Arthritis Center, http://www.hopkins-arthritis.org/patient-corner/disease-management/depression.htm.

3. James L. Henry, "The Need for Knowledge Translation in Chronic Pain," *Pain Research and Management* 3, no. 6 (2008), 468.

4. Carol Jay Levy, *A Pained Life* (Xlibris Corporation, 2003), 317.

5. Arthur W. Frank, *The Wounded Storyteller: Body, Illness, and Ethics* (Chicago: University of Chicago Press, 1995), 77–96.

6. Mary Carmichael, "The Changing Science of Pain," *Newsweek,* June 4, 2007, 43.

7. Theoretical physicist David Bohm, in *Wholeness and the Implicate Order* (Boston: Routledge and Kegan Paul, 1980), 21–22, notes how, before the rise of seventeenth-century science, to "measure" something meant to understand its "innermost being," the totality of its inner proportions. A measure was a form of insight gained, not by conforming to external standards, but by creative insight and understanding of the deeper meaning of the structures and proportions of that which one wished to understand.

8. Arthur Rosenfeld, *The Truth about Chronic Pain* (New York: Basic Books, 2003).

9. Marni Jackson, *Pain, the Science and Culture of Why We Hurt* (Toronto: Vintage Canada, 2002).

10. David B. Morris, *The Culture of Pain* (Berkeley: University of California Press, 1991), 72–74.

11. Eric J. Cassell, *The Nature of Suffering and the Goals of Medicine* (New York: Oxford University Press), 57.

12. Ross A. Hauser, *Prolo Your Pain Away!* (Oak Park, Ill: Beulah Land Press, 1998).

2. That Which Has No Words, That Which Cannot Be Seen

1. David B. Morris, *The Culture of Pain* (Berkeley: University of California Press, 1991), 67.

2. "The Poetry Symposium," *New York Times Book Review,* November 21, 2004, 13.

3. David Kuhl, *What Dying People Want: Practical Wisdom for the End of Life* (Scarborough, ON: Doubleday Canada, 2002), 94.

4. Morris, *Culture of Pain,* 244.

5. Alphonse Daudet, *In the Land of Pain,* ed. and trans. Julian Barnes (New York: Alfred A. Knopf, 2002), 15.

6. Julian Barnes, introduction to *Land of Pain,* v.

7. Daudet, *Land of Pain,* 45, 47.

8. Elaine Scarry, *The Body in Pain: The Making and Unmaking of the World* (New York: Oxford University Press, 1985), 4.

9. Angela Mailis-Gagnon and David Israelson, *Beyond Pain: Making the Mind-Body Connection* (Toronto: Viking Canada, 2003).

10. Chester Buckenmaier, "Battlefield Medicine and Combat Trauma: New Approaches to Pain Relief," American Pain Foundation, September 9, 2005, http://www.painfoundation.org/page.asp?file=ManageYourPain/Chats/Veterans090905.htm.

11. Canadian Consortium on Pain Mechanisms Diagnosis and Management, Network Program, Final Report: Market Analysis, http://www.fhs.mcmaster.ca/paininstitute/.

12. Marni Jackson, *Pain: The Science and Culture of Why We Hurt* (Toronto: Vintage Canada, 2002), 144.

13. Scott Fishman, *The War on Pain,* with Lisa Berger (New York: Quill, 2001), 85–87.

14. Arthur Rosenfeld, *The Truth about Chronic Pain* (New York: Basic Books, 2003), 12.

3. Pain and the Self

1. Scott Fishman, *The War on Pain,* with Lisa Berger (New York: Quill, 2001), 94.

2. Melanie Thernstrom, "Pain, the Disease," *New York Times,* December 16, 2001, 66.

3. Fishman, *War on Pain,* 62.

4. Arthur Rosenfeld, *The Truth about Chronic Pain* (New York: Basic Books, 2003), 109.

5. Arthur W. Frank, *The Wounded Storyteller: Body, Illness, and Ethics* (Chicago: University of Chicago Press, 1995), xii.

6. David B. Morris, *The Culture of Pain* (Berkeley: University of California Press, 1991), 71.

7. Angela Mailis-Gagnon and David Israelson, *Beyond Pain: Making the Mind-Body Connection* (Toronto: Viking Canada, 2003), 197.

8. James L. Henry, "The Need for Knowledge Translation in Chronic Pain," *Pain Research and Management* 3, no. 6 (2008), 469.

9. Elaine Scarry, *The Body in Pain: The Making and Unmaking of the World* (New York: Alfred A. Knopf, 2002), 31.

10. David Kuhl, *What Dying People Want: Practical Wisdom for the End of Life* (Scarborough, ON: Doubleday Canada, 2002), 93.

11. Marni Jackson, *Pain: The Science and Culture of Why We Hurt* (Toronto: Vintage Canada, 2002), 160.

12. Scarry, *Body in Pain,* 32–33.

13. Jon Kabat-Zinn, *Coming to Our Senses: Healing Ourselves and the World through Mindfulness* (New York, Hyperion, 2005), 88.

14. Ibid., 89.

15. Arthur Frank, *The Renewal of Generosity: Illness, Medicine, and How to Live* (Chicago: University of Chicago Press, 2004), 72.

16. Emily Dickinson, *The Complete Poems of Emily Dickinson* (Boston: Little, Brown, 1924), pt. 1, no. 19.

17. Eric J. Cassell, *The Nature of Suffering and the Goals of Medicine* (New York: Oxford University Press, 1991), 36.

18. Balfour Mount, "The Culture of Pain," CBC *Ideas,* September 22–26, 2003, 48.

19. John O'Donohue, *Beauty: The Invisible Embrace* (New York: HarperCollins, 2004), 13.

20. Ibid., 23.

21. Ibid., 66–67.

22. Jon Kabat-Zinn, *Full Catastrophe Living: Using the Wisdom of Your Body and Mind to Face Stress, Pain, and Illness* (New York: Delta, 1990).

4. Pain and the World of Pain Management

1. Scott Fishman, *The War on Pain,* with Lisa Berger (New York: Quill, 2001) xi.

2. Arthur Rosenfeld, *The Truth about Chronic Pain.* (New York: Basic Books, 2003), 268.

3. David B. Morris, *The Culture of Pain.* (Berkeley: University of California Press, 1991), 67.

4. Barry Sessle, president of the Canadian Pain Society, in the CPS Winter 2008 newsletter cites data showing that 67.5% of over forty health-care professional schools in Canada have no formal pain content in their curriculum. Veterinary medicine devotes eighty-seven hours to pain, human medicine only sixteen hours. Key proceedings of the roundtable discussion of pain-management professionals held by the APF in April 2008 (Provider Prescribing Patterns and Perceptions: Identifying Solutions to Build Consensus on Opiod Use in Pain Management) called for a coordinated effort to require pain-management training to be part of the core curriculums at U.S. Schools of Medicine, Nursing, and Pharmacy.

5. Fishman, *War on Pain,* 257.

6. Rosenfeld, *Truth,* 289.

7. Atul Gawande, *Complications: A Surgeon's Notes on an Imperfect Science.* (New York: Henry Holt, 2003), 118.

8. Marni Jackson, *Pain, the Science and Culture of Why We Hurt.* (Toronto: Vintage Canada, 2002), 36.

9. Michael Stein, *The Lonely Patient: How We Experience Illness.* (New York: William Morrow, 2007), 20.

10. Angela Mailis-Gagnon and David Israelson, *Beyond Pain: Making the Mind-Body Connection.* (Toronto: Vintage Canada, 2002).

11. Sara Cassidy, "Pharma Buster," *Focus: Victoria's Monthly Magazine of People, Ideas and Culture,* September 2005, 26.

12. Stephen S. Hall, "The Drug Lords," *New York Times,* November 14, 2004, 6–7.

13. Jerome Groopman, "When Pain Remains," *New Yorker,* October 10, 2005, 36–41.

14. Morris, *Culture,* 156.

15. Nellie A. Radomsky, *Lost Voices: Women, Chronic Pain, and Abuse.* (Philadelphia: Haworth Press, 1995), 138.

16. Morris, *Culture,* 70.

17. "The Culture of Pain," CBC *Ideas*, September 22–26, 2003, 5.

18. Ibid., 5.

19. Eric J. Cassell, *The Nature of Suffering and the Goals of Medicine.* (New York: Oxford University Press, 1991), 233.

20. Stein, *Lonely Patient*, 5.

21. Cassell, *Suffering*, 31, 247.

22. Gawande, *Complications*, 118.

23. Arthur W. Frank, *The Renewal of Generosity: Illness, Medicine, and How to Live.* (Chicago: University of Chicago Press, 2004), 1.

24. David Kuhl, *What Dying People Want: Practical Wisdom for the End of Life.* (Scarborough, ON: Doubleday Canada, 2002), 99–100.

25. Kuhl, *Dying People*, 114.

26. Ibid., 155.

27. Stein, *Lonely Patient*, 203.

28. Steven Aung, "Loving Kindness: The Most Powerful Healing Energy," Association of Complementary Physicians of British Columbia Newsletter, Spring 2002, 1, 5.

29. Cassell, *Suffering*, 23.

30. Jan Hoffman, "Doctors' Delicate Balance in Keeping Hope Alive," *New York Times*, December 24, 2005.

31. Kuhl, *Dying People*, 295.

32. Atul Gawande, *Better: A Surgeon's Notes on Performance.* (New York: Henry Holt, 2007), 161.

33. Frank, *Generosity*, 18, 83.

34. Nathan Thornburgh, "Teaching Doctors to Care," *Time*, June 19, 2006, Canadian edition, 47.

5. Pain Medicine

1. Frank Owen, "The DEA's War on Pain Doctors," *Pain Relief Network*, November 5, 2003, 4, http://www.painreliefnetwork.org/prn/the-deas-war-on-pain-doctors.php.

2. David B. Morris, *The Culture of Pain* (Berkeley: University of California Press, 1991), 191.

3. Ronald T. Libby, "Treating Doctors as Drug Dealers: The DEA's War on Prescription Painkillers," Policy Analysis no. 545, CATO Institute, June 16, 2005, 1.

4. Scott Fishman, *The War on Pain*, with Lisa Berger (New York: Quill, 2001), 186.

5. "Addiction, Physical Dependency, Tolerance: Confused?" Newsletter of the American Pain Foundation, Summer 2003, 1.

6. "Pain Patient Finds Relief," Newsletter of the American Pain Foundation, Summer 2003, 2.

7. Elizabeth Enright, "Rooting out Pain," *The Magazine*, AARP, September/October 2004.

8. Fishman, *War on Pain*, 127.

9. Marni Jackson, *Pain: The Science and Culture of Why We Hurt* (Toronto: Vintage Canada, 2002), 255, 288.

10. Fishman, *War on Pain*, 186.

11. Ibid., 184.

12. Alphonse Daudet, *In the Land of Pain*, ed. and trans. Julian Barnes (New York: Alfred. A. Knopf, 2002), 43. Daudet's emphasis.

13. Arthur Rosenfeld, *The Truth about Chronic Pain* (New York: Basic Books, 2003).

14. Michael Stein, *The Lonely Patient: How We Experience Illness* (New York: William Morrow, 2007), 52.

15. Jon Kabat-Zinn, *Full Catastrophe Living: Using the Wisdom of Your Body and Mind to Face Stress, Pain, and Illness* (New York: Delta, 1990), 228, 291.

16. Mary Carmichael, "The Changing Science of Pain," *Newsweek*, June 4, 2007, 46.

17. Nanette Gartell, "A Doctor's Toxic Shock," *New York Times Magazine*, section 6, January 4, 2004, 58.

18. Stephen S. Hall, "The Drug Lords," *New York Times Book Review*, November 14, 2004, 9; Marcia Angell, *The Truth about the Drug Companies: How They Deceive Us and What to Do About It* (New York: Random House, 2005); Jerry Avorn, *Powerful Medicines: The Benefits, Risks, and Costs of Prescription Drugs* (New York: Alfred A. Knopf, 2004). See also Ray Moynihan and Alan Cassels, *Selling Sickness: How the World's Biggest Pharmaceutical Companies Are Turning Us All into Patients* (Vancouver: Greystone Books, 2005).

19. See, for instance, Neil Osterweil, "What a Pain! Now It's Tylenol Troubles," *Medpage Today*, http://medpagetoday.com/tbprint.cfm?tbid=974; and Heather Simonsen, "Hidden Risk: Tylenol Ingredient Can Be Dangerous," *Salt Lake Tribune*, May 3, 2006.

20. National Center for Complementary and Alternative Medicine, National Institutes of Health, http://nccam.nih.gov/health/whatiscam/.

21. Herbert Benson, Julie Corliss, and Geoffrey Cowley, "Brain Check," *Newsweek*, September 27, 2004, 46.

22. Ibid., 47.

23. Chester Buckenmaier, "Battlefield Medicine and Combat Trauma: New Approaches to Pain Relief," American Pain Foundation, September 9, 2005, http://www.painfounda tion.org/page.asp?file=ManageYourPain/Chats/Veterans090905.htm.

6. On Science and Time

1. See, e.g., Robert G. Klein et al., "A Randomized Double-Blind Trial of Dextrose-Glycerine-Phenol Injections for Chronic, Low Back Pain," *Journal of Spinal Disorders* (1993), 23–33; and Kenneth D. Reeves and Khatab Hassanein, "Randomized Prospective Double-Blind Placebo-Controlled Study of Dextrose Prolotherapy for Knee Osteoarthritis with or without ACL Laxity," *Alternative Therapies* (2000), 68–80.

2. Eric Cassell, *The Nature of Suffering and the Goals of Medicine* (New York: Oxford University Press, 1991), 235.

3. Marni Jackson, *Pain, the Science and Culture of Why We Hurt* (Toronto: Vintage Canada, 2002), 46.

4. Ibid., 121–22.

5. David Leonhardt, "Why Doctors So Often Get It Wrong," *New York Times*, February 22, 2006, Business section.

6. Melanie Thernstrom, "Pain, the Disease," *New York Times*, December 16, 2001.

7. Scott Fishman, *The War on Pain*, with Lisa Berger (New York: Quill: 2001), esp. chap. 5.

8. David B. Morris, *The Culture of Pain* (Berkeley: University of California Press, 1991), 67, 70.

9. Fishman, *War on Pain*, 57.

10. Ibid., 80.

11. Ibid., 87.

12. Arthur W. Frank, *The Renewal of Generosity: Illness, Medicine, and How to Live* (Chicago: University of Chicago Press, 2004), 44.

13. Nellie A. Radomsky, *Lost Voices: Women, Chronic Pain, and Abuse* (Philadelphia: Haworth Press, 1995).

14. Peter Salgo, "The Doctor Will See You for Exactly Seven Minutes," *New York Times,* March 22, 2006, Op-Ed.

15. Milt Freudenheim, "Trying to Save by Increasing Doctors' Fees," *New York Times,* July 21, 2008, Business section.

7. Pain and Others

1. Richard Payne, "Hurting While Black: Racially Based Disparities in Pain Care," Newsletter of the American Pain Foundation, Summer 2003, 5.

2. American Pain Society, "Racial and Ethnic Identifiers in Pain Management: The Importance to Research, Clinical Practice, and Public Health Policy," October 22, 2004, http://www.ampainsoc.org/advocacy/ethnoracial.htm.

3. Sheri Hall, "The Pain Gap: Minorities in America Are Considered 'Under Treated' for Their Pain from Medical Conditions," Asbury Park Press, March 15, 2005.

4. Angela Mailis-Gagnon, "Calling All Those Interested in Pain and Culture," Newsletter, Canadian Pain Society, Summer 2008.

5. Diane E. Hoffmann and Anita J. Tarzian, "The Girl Who Cried Pain: A Bias against Women in the Treatment of Pain," *Journal of Law, Medicine and Ethics,* 29 (2001).

6. David B. Morris, *The Culture of Pain* (Berkeley: University of California Press, 1991), 67.

7. Arthur Rosenfeld, *The Truth about Pain* (New York: Basic Books, 2003), 266.

8. Marni Jackson, *Pain: The Science and Culture of Why We Hurt* (Toronto: Vintage Canada, 2002), 34, 39–40.

9. Hermione Lee, introduction to *On Being Ill,* by Virginia Woolf (Ashfield, MA.: Paris Press, 2002), xxvi.

10. Eric J. Cassell, *The Nature of Suffering and the Goals of Medicine* (New York: Oxford University Press, 1991), 63.

11. Scott Fishman, *The War on Pain,* with Lisa Berger (New York: Quill, 2001), 94.

12. Miriam Greenspan, *Healing through the Dark Emotions: The Wisdom of Grief, Fear, and Despair* (Boston: Shambhala, 2003), 128.

13. David Kuhl, *What Dying People Want: Practical Wisdom for the End of Life* (Scarborough, ON: Doubleday Canada, 2002), 56.

14. Morris, *Culture,* 245.

15. Fishman, *War on Pain.*

16. *Monday Magazine,* Victoria, BC, May 13–19, 2004, Letters.

17. Cassell, *Suffering,* 246–47.

18. Virginia Woolf, *On Being Ill* (Ashfield, MA: Paris Press, 2002), 9–10, 15–16.

19. Michael Stein, *The Lonely Patient: How We Experience Illness* (New York: William Morrow, 2007), 58.

8. Where Are We with Chronic Pain? A Patient's Perspective

1. Ronald Dubner, "Redefining the Search for the Magic Bullet," *The Scientist,* March 28, 2005, 2, http://www.the-scientist.com/2005/03/28/S12/1.

2. Claudia Wallis, "The Right (and Wrong) Way to Treat Pain," *Time,* February 28, 2005, 37, Canadian edition.

3. Jane E. Brody, "Injections to Kick-Start Tissue Repair," *New York Times,* August 7, 2007, Health section.

4. Wallis, *Time,* 43.

5. Ronald T. Libby, "Treating Doctors as Drug Dealers: The DEA's War on Prescription Painkillers," Policy Analysis no. 545, CATO Institute, June 16, 2005, 2.

6. American Pain Foundation, "Provider Prescribing Patterns and Perceptions: Identifying Solutions to Build Consensus on Opioid Use in Pain Management—A Roundtable Discussion," Key Proceedings, April 2008, 9.

7. Roman D. Jovey, President's Note, Canadian Pain Society Newsletter, Winter 2006, 2.

8. Anne McIlroy, "Solve this Agony," *Globe and Mail,* October 21, 2006, Science section.

9. Dionne Brand, *No Language Is Neutral* (Toronto: Coach House Press, 1990), 31.

10. Wallis, *Time,* 34.

11. Canadian Pain Coalition, "National Pain Awareness Week Puts Focus on the Epidemic of Pain in Canada," *Health Care News for South West Ontario,* 1, http://www.the healthline.ca/viewnews.asp?newsid=497.

12. Holly Lake, "Take Charge of Pain: A Life of Pain, Day 5," *Ottawa Sun,* October 20, 2005.

13. Arthur W. Frank, *The Wounded Storyteller: Body, Illness, and Ethics* (Chicago: University of Chicago Press, 1995), 25.

14. "Lawmakers Discuss Treatment of Chronic Pain," *World Now,* July 18, 2005, http://www.wlns.com/global/story.asp?s=3465023&ClientType=Print.

Index

About the Authors

Lous Heshusius was a professor of education for twenty years at the University of Northern Iowa and at York University in Toronto before a catastrophic car accident in 1996 changed her life forever. Previously, she was a school teacher in the Netherlands, where she was born, and in the United States. She has also been a visiting professor at universities in the United States, Canada, and New Zealand. She has published numerous articles, written and edited three books in the areas of critical special education and educational research, and is the recipient of a lifetime achievement award given by the conference committee of the Annual Conference on Disability Studies and Education. On long-term disability leave because of ongoing pain, she now lives quietly in the countryside with her cats at the edge of Victoria, British Columbia. She has two daughters.

Dr. Scott M. Fishman is Chief of the Division of Pain Medicine and Professor of Anesthesiology and Pain Medicine at the University of California, Davis, and President of the American Pain Foundation. He was formerly Medical Director of the Massachusetts General Hospital Pain Center at Harvard Medical School. His recent books include *The War on Pain* (2001) and *Listening to Pain* (2006) as well as two coauthored books—*The Massachusetts General Hospital Handbook of Pain Management* (2002) and *Essentials of Pain Medicine and Regional Anesthesia*. He is also senior editor of the journal *Pain Medicine*. Dr. Fishman lectures on all aspects of pain and its treatment throughout the United States and is a frequent source of information for the media. He has appeared on such television programs as the *Today Show, Good Morning America,* and *ABC Nightly News,* served as the pain expert for Discoveryhealth.com, and has a monthly question-and-answer column for the American Pain Foundation newsletter.

David B. Morris is a writer, scholar, and professor at the University of Virginia. He has written numerous essays and two prize-winning books on British literature—*The Religious Sublime* (1972) and *Alexander Pope: The Genius of Sense* (1984). *The Culture of Pain* (1991) won a prestigious PEN prize. He has subsequently addressed numerous medical groups and in 1999 served as Gunn-Loke Lecturer at the University of Washington Multidisciplinary Pain Center. In 2000 he delivered a plenary lecture at the Tenth World Congress on Pain, and in 2005 he co-edited, with distinguished pain specialists John D. Loeser and Daniel B. Carr, *Narrative, Pain, and Suffering* (published by the International Association for the Study of Pain). His recent books include *Illness and Culture in the Postmodern Age* (1998), which describes some of the ways we are coming to understand illness as always constructed at the crossroads of biology and culture.